Paediatric Cariology

Quintessentials of Dental Practice – 14
Paediatric Dentistry/Orthodontics - 2

Paediatric Cariology

By
Marie Thérèse Hosey
Christopher Deery
Paula Jane Waterhouse

Editor-in-Chief: Nairn H F Wilson
Editor Paediatric Dentistry/Orthodontics: Marie Thérèse Hosey

Quintessence Publishing Co. Ltd.

London, Berlin, Chicago, Paris, Milan, Barcelona, Istanbul
São Paulo, Tokyo, New Delhi, Moscow, Prague, Warsaw

British Library Cataloguing-in Publication Data

Deery, C.
  Paediatric cariology - (Quintessentials of dental practice;
  14. Paediatric dentistry/orthodontics; 2)
  1. Dental caries in children - Treatment
  I. Title II. Hosey, Marie-Therese Wilson, III.Waterhouse, P.J.
  617.6´7´0083

ISBN 1850970734

ISBN 1-85097-073-4

Foreword

It is very sad that so many children continue to suffer the ravages of dental caries and are faced with the prospect of dental interventions, possibly including one or more general anaesthetics, at a young age. Indeed, it is very sad that many more children are not caries-free, given that caries is a preventable disease.

Paediatric Cariology is an excellent addition to the rapidly expanding Quintessentials of Dental Practice series. Understanding, preventing and, in particular, managing caries in children may not be viewed by some as one of the more glamorous aspect of the clinical practice of dentistry but, if done well, is widely accepted to be one of the most rewarding. More often than not, the challenge is to deal with at least three things at one and the same time – the child as the patient, the caries and the parent who may be anxious, guilt-ridden or, in the more difficult cases, indifferent. Not an easy task, but one that can be simplified if familiar with the latest thinking and clinical guidance as contained in this most helpful, easy-to-read, well illustrated book.

As has come to be expected of books in the Quintessentials of Dental Practice series, the focus, as in the present book, is on up-to-date knowledge and understanding of immediate practical relevance. This book fulfils this expectation and, as such, may be used to great benefit in the care of children. Paediatric dentistry has changed a great deal in recent years and is set to change further with the increasing use of alternative materials and techniques and attainable improvements in the oral health of children. *Paediatric cariology* is an aspect of clinical practice that practitioners need to keep informed on. This book provides the ideal means to meet this need.

Nairn Wilson
Editor-in Chief

Preface

Managing caries in children is a challenge to every dentist. The aim of management for every dental team is to provide care, which helps a child to become dentally aware, avoid iatrogenic damage and to grow to be a fit young adult with healthy teeth. This is principally achieved by empowering the child and their carer with preventive advice so that they value dental health and know how to maintain it.

The prevention of dental caries is always the first priority in paediatric dental care and this involves the whole dental team, often supported by community health improvement initiatives, especially water fluoridation.

Unfortunately, when caries occurs in the primary dentition the morphology of the primary molars, in particular, leads to early pulpal involvement. Therefore, early diagnosis, although often difficult, is important to simplify treatment. Luckily, pulp therapies and preformed crowns are relatively easy to perform and the addition of these techniques to the dental therapist armamentarium is a great asset to the dental team in the UK.

We hope that this book will, firstly, inspire better routine preventative care and, secondly, provide dental operators (dentists and therapists alike) with the modern diagnostic tools and restorative techniques to manage caries in children in primary care dentistry in the UK.

Acknowledgements

We express our gratitude to Dr Howard Moody, Dr Chris Longbottom and Mr Toby Gilgrass for supplying some of the photographic images. Thanks to Hazel, Ed and Richard – our long-suffering spouses – for all your support during the preparation of this book.

Contents

Chapter 1
Paediatric Cariology: Management and Myth

Aim

This chapter aims to emphasise the importance of the management of caries in children in respect of their continued dental, emotional and educational development. In addition, various myths surrounding paediatric cariology will be discussed.

Outcome

Upon reading this chapter, the practitioner should have gained an understanding of the importance of ensuring that children remain free of both acute and chronic dental pain and appreciate the contribution of the primary dentition, in particular, to overall health and development. The dental team should also be familiar with the chronology of the development of the dentition and appreciate how knowledge of this assists in determining the effect of common childhood illnesses upon the dental hard tissues.

Introduction

Dental caries is one of the most prevalent of human diseases. This disease involves the mineralised tissues of the teeth, namely enamel, dentine and cementum, caused by the action of microorganisms on fermentable carbohydrates. It is characterised by demineralisation of the mineral portion of these tissues followed by the disintegration of their organic material. The disease can result in bacterial invasion and death of the pulp and the spread of infection into the periapical tissues, causing pain. In its early stages, however, the disease can be arrested since it is possible for remineralisation to occur.Over recent years there has been a decline in the prevalence of caries in the Western World. Possible reasons for this include the widespread use of fluoride (especially in toothpaste), changes in the diet, the increased use of antibiotics, and possible changes in the virulence of microorganisms.

The decline in caries prevalence has been greatest on the smooth surfaces of teeth. The pit and fissured surfaces of the molar teeth now have the greatest

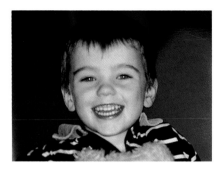

Fig 1-1 A visit to the dentist should be a pleasant experience.

disease susceptibility, although buccal and palatal pits and fissures remain caries prone. The decline in caries, however, has not been uniform but skewed. The Scottish Health Boards' Dental Epidemiological Programme survey carried out in 1992/93 showed caries in 7% of 12-year-old children.

Unfortunately, many dental practitioners do not see the value in restoring the primary dentition. This reinforces the view of many parents that primary teeth are expendable. We hope that this book will encourage dentists, dental therapists and hygienists to develop their skills to meet the challenge of treating the young child and promote a change in attitude in those who do not value the primary dentition (Fig 1-1).

So Why Should We Restore the Primary Dentition?

It is becoming increasingly clear that dental health is intertwined with general health and development. Pain and infection have a detrimental effect on health. These are obvious in the child with acute pain, but chronic toothache also causes problems. A child with chronic dental pain cannot thrive and all carious teeth are likely to cause pain and sensitivity from time to time, resulting in:
- loss of sleep
- mood, behaviour changes and poor concentration
- uncomfortable eating, with subsequent loss of appetite and failure to meet developmental milestones: height, weight and head (brain) circumference.

Therefore, the child with dental caries may not thrive physically, emotionally or intellectually, compared to the caries-free child (Figs 1-2 to 1-4). Where children are concerned, their medical, and particularly dental, well-being is of paramount importance. Even relatively simple dental problems can impact upon the medical or educational needs of children, especially on those already diagnosed with medical disorders or learning disabilities.

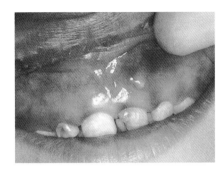

Fig 1-2 Young child with carious upper incisors and an abscess on tooth 51.

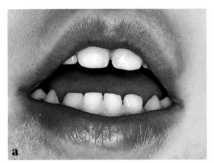

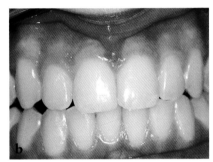

Fig 1-3 Caries-free child with (a) primary teeth and (b) permanent teeth.

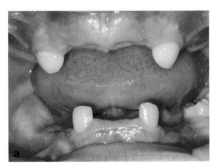

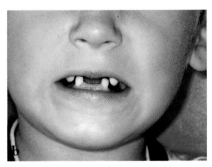

Fig 1-4 Child who has had multiple teeth extracted (a) intra-oral view and (b) extra-oral view.

The dental practitioner should aim to motivate the patient and their family by demonstrating that teeth are not disposable and restore primary dentition because it helps:
- restore form
- restore aesthetics

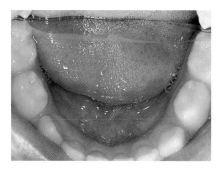

Fig 1-5 Primary teeth act as a natural space maintainer for the permanent teeth.

- restore function (mastication and speech)
- maintain space for the permanent teeth (Fig 1-5)
- acclimatisation
- avoid pain and sepsis — avoid damage to the permanent teeth
- avoid extraction, particularly under general anaesthesia
- avoid sepsis and surgical intervention in the medically compromised child.

The Chronology of the Development of the Dentition

The development of the primary and permanent dentitions is affected by:
- genetic factors
- nutrition
- somatic growth and development.

There is little variation reported between different races in the timing of eruption of the primary dentition. Racial variation, however, can be seen in the eruption of the permanent dentition — for example, Asian children complete their dental development faster that their Caucasian peers. Therefore, care must be applied when dentists seek to compare an individual child to the "normal" eruption times (Table 1-1).

Studies in Peru, on malnourished children, have shown that infants were delayed in the eruption of their primary teeth. This link between nutrition, dental development and general growth can also be seen in premature and low birthweight babies. These babies will "catch-up" on their dental development once their nutrition and medical problem has been rectified and somatic growth will "catch up" with the normal milestones for length, weight and head circumference.

Table 1-1 **Eruption dates of primary teeth and secondary teeth**

Primary Teeth	Eruption Time (Months)
Central incisor	6
Lateral incisor	9
Canine	18
First molar	12
Second molar	24

Calcification commences 4-6 months *in-utero*
Root formation complete 12-18 months after eruption

Secondary Teeth	Eruption Time (Years)	Calcification Starts (Years)
Central incisors	7	0.3
Lateral incisors	8	0.3/1★
Canine	9 /12★	0.3
First premolar	10	2
Second premolar	11	2
First molar	6	Birth
Second molar	12	3
Third molar	16-24	8-14

★lower/upper
  Root formation complete 2-3 years after eruption

A nutritionist often investigates children who fail to meet their normal developmental milestones. Such children may be placed on dietary supplements: these are generally carbohydrate-rich and so oral hygiene and fluoride therapy are of paramount importance. Other children are referred for dental care to manage dental pain, which may be deterring adequate food intake.

The dental team plays a key role in infant growth and development.

Childhood Fever and Caries Susceptibility

Common childhood illnesses can affect the coincidental dental hard-tissue formation. This can result in hypomineralisation and discolouration. As soon as this is diagnosed, the dental team should be alerted to the fact that the child will have a *high caries risk* and consequently needs personalised, enhanced preventive management.

Teeth affected by childhood fevers have increased susceptibility to dental caries due to:
- altered tooth morphology
- enamel porosity
- difficulties in maintaining good oral hygiene due to sensitivity.

An example of this is molar incisor hypomineralisation (MIH), in which the permanent incisors and first permanent molars are affected (and possibly also the tips of the canines). The affected teeth appear to be prone to post-eruptive enamel loss.

Examples of the common childhood illnesses that can cause enamel defects are:
- chickenpox
- measles
- middle ear infections
- fevers caused by respiratory or urinary tract infections
- other fevers that cause skin rashes (remember that enamel and skin share a common ectodermal origin).

Myths

Calcium Deficiency
- The body regulates calcium levels so rigorously that deficiency in the developed world is rare.
- Calcium deficiency does not lead to calcium "leaking" back out of the teeth.
- Once enamel is formed, the only reason calcium is lost is due to an environmental cause such as caries or acid erosion or attrition.

Breastfeeding and Teeth?
- Breastfeeding **IS** highly recommended.
- Human milk **IS** better than cows' milk for human babies.

- Breastfeeding assists growth and is especially beneficial to brain development.
- Provided children are weaned at the normal time there is **NO** damage to teeth.
- **BUT** breastfeeding on demand, especially during the night, beyond weaning, **DOES** cause caries.

Do "Soft" Teeth Run in the Family?
Inherited defects
Children with congenital enamel defects such as amelogenesis imperfecta or disease of the other dental hard tissues (e.g. dentinogenesis imperfecta) may be more susceptible to caries, but these conditions are rare.

- A family history (pedigree) should be ascertained if a congenital defect of the dental hard tissues is suspected.
- Exfoliated or extracted teeth can be examined microscopically.
- Environmental causes (i.e., the effect of a common childhood illness) should be ruled out first.

"Family" caries
- Families **DO** tend to pass on their dietary habits through generations. Therefore, granny losing her teeth early could be an indication of a "sweet tooth" being a family phenomenon.
- *Streptococcus mutans*, the main pathogen responsible for caries, **IS** transmissible and there is very good evidence to show that it is passed from mother to baby.
- Children of mothers with a high caries rate are more likely to develop caries themselves.

Medicine
- Medicines, in particular, elixirs, **CAN** cause caries **BUT** only if they contain sugar.
- Some medicines are sucrose-free, but may contain other sugars such as glucose syrup.
- "Sugars-free" means no sugar at all.
- Many paediatric medicines including antibiotics **ARE** now available in "sugars-free" preparations. Dentists and their teams should advise parents and medical and pharmacy colleagues to add the letters 'SF' for sugars-free to written prescriptions — this is particularly important in cases in which repeat prescriptions are required.
- Antibiotics **DO NOT** cause discolouration or hypomineralisation leading to increased caries susceptibility; it was the illness for which antibi-

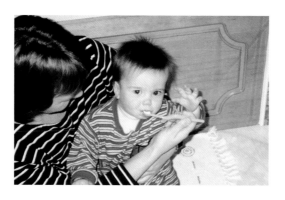

Fig 1-6 Start early.

otics were prescribed that was the culprit. However, ensure sugars-free antibiotics are prescribed in future.

- Doctors rarely prescribe tetracyclines to children, only in exceptional circumstances (e.g. cystic fibrosis).

Practical Tips

- If good dental health habits have been established in infancy, caries in the permanent teeth is less likely (Fig 1-6).
- A child with chronic toothache can fail to thrive, so dental disease needs to be treated.
- If caries is left untreated the parent must be informed of this and be in agreement (e.g. a tooth that is soon to exfoliate).

Chapter 2
Diagnosis of Dental Caries

Aim

This chapter aims to update the principles of caries detection, diagnosis and record-keeping, and to give guidance on the appropriate use of adjuncts to caries diagnosis in the child and adolescent.

Outcome

On reading this chapter, the practitioner should feel more confident in caries diagnosis, especially in respect to the examination and caries risk assessment of children and be familiar with the relevant supporting theories in modern cariology.

Introduction

All children and adolescents are individuals and, as such, their dental care should be customised to their specific needs. The first stage in this process is to take a history (dental, social and medical) and complete a careful examination. The history and examination should be thorough and recorded in a systematic way, in order to gather all the available information and avoid omissions. The history must also be appropriate to the age of the child — for example, with older children it is important to take the child's views into account, even at the expense of those of their parents or carers. The key to success is to get off on the right foot and gain the child's trust and the parent's confidence. Therefore, the initial greeting of the child and their carers is critical (Fig 2-1).

The First Visit

A brief history of dental attendance should be recorded, as should the current complaint (if any). It is important that the family is made to feel welcome when they attend for care. Any implied criticism of past behaviour is likely to have a detrimental effect on future behaviour. In simple terms, child patients won't wish to return for treatment or will be less compliant if they

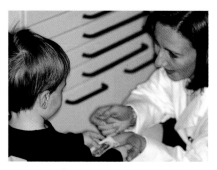

Fig 2-1 The initial greeting of the child is paramount.

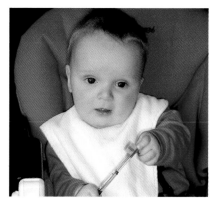

Fig 2-2 Dental care is needed as soon as the first teeth erupt.

think they will be "told off". History-taking helps with the assessment of the families' attitudes to dental health and caries risk assessment (Fig 2-2).

A brief history of previous dental care is invaluable. For example, it is useful to know how well the child coped with the provision of previous restorations and local anaesthesia. The use of local anaesthesia is also an indication of the quality and prognosis of existing restorations. Such information can help with assessing the child's ability to cope with any proposed treatment.

Examination

While talking to the child, it should quickly become apparent how agreeable to examination and treatment they are likely to be. The subsequent stages of the examination can then be tailored to the patient's ability to cooperate. It may be that only a brief examination will be possible at the initial consultation.

Extra-oral Examination
- Check general appearance
- Demeanour
- Swelling
- Asymmetry
- Lymphadenopathy
- Skeletal pattern.

Intra-oral Examination
- Soft tissues
- Periodontal tissues
- Plaque levels (oral hygiene)
- Gingival bleeding (as well as being indicative of gingivitis, may indicate active approximal caries)
- Teeth:
    - caries diagnosis
    - hypoplasia/opacities
- Occlusion.

Caries Risk Assessment

A key element of the examination of a patient is the caries risk assessment. The results of this assessment should be recorded in the notes, as a patient-specific prompt, to encourage appropriate preventive management, such as the provision of fissure sealants. The recording of caries risk will also promote best practice by assisting with clinical audit.

Caries risk assessment is not a new concept to most dentists; it is something most dentists do implicitly for all patients. The step that is more novel is to make this an explicit action.

Previous Disease
Past behaviour and disease experience are one of the best predictors of future disease. Therefore, predictors of high caries activity are:
- The presence of restorations
- Previous extractions
- New disease.

Dietary Factors
- Non-intrinsic non-milk sugars in the diet cause caries.
- Patients whose diet is high in such sugars, and particularly when these products are consumed frequently, are likely to be of high caries risk.
- Time of consumption is also important:
    - access to any sugar at night increases caries risk,
    - milk can cause caries if a child is given free access at night, when the anti-caries benefits of saliva are reduced,
    - access to a sugary snack within an hour of bedtime in a young child is associated with increased caries risk.

Social Factors

Like heart disease and cancer, caries is a socio-economic disease. Therefore, in broad terms, the patient's area post code helps predict their caries risk. For better management it is helpful to find out:

- Who cares for the child?
- How easy is it for them to attend?
- Information about siblings, interests and pets helps with behaviour management by making the child feel special.
- School performance might highlight a learning disability.

Fluoride Use and Plaque Control

- The use of fluoride toothpaste is largely responsible for the reduction in caries prevalence seen in the Western World over the past 30 years.
- Oral hygiene as a measure of the frequency and effectiveness of toothbrushing (assuming a fluoride toothpaste is used) is therefore an important factor.
- For those lucky enough to be living in fluoridated areas or with a history of use of fluoride supplements this must be included in an assessment.

Medical History

Medical history may influence caries risk in a number of ways:

- A condition that predisposes to caries (e.g. xerostomia during chemotherapy).
- A condition where the consequences of caries (either its treatment or sepsis) can be a threat to the patient (e.g. those at risk of infective endocarditis).
- A condition that confers reduced ability to cooperate with dental care or to perform oral health procedures (e.g. cerebral palsy).

Saliva

Saliva plays a pivotal role in the prevention of caries, as it contains both specific and non-specific antibacterial agents such as IgA, lysozyme and lactoferrin. It buffers acids and maintains the oral pH. A reduction in the production of saliva will therefore increase an individual's caries risk. There is considerable individual variation in the quality of saliva, and although tests for the constituents of saliva and buffering capacity exist, these have a limited role at the chairside at present. However, if a dentist suspects a reduction in salivary flow this would influence a caries risk assessment.

Bacteria

Streptococcus mutans and *Lactobacillus* levels correlate with caries risk at a population level. Unfortunately, the levels of these bacteria are not predictive at an individual level.

Fissure Shape
Fissure shape is not a good predictor of caries risk. The identification of caries predilection sites, which includes the occlusal fissures of the permanent molars, does play an important role in caries diagnosis and prevention, but a clinician cannot reliably tell the depth or, more importantly, the shape of a fissure.

The Dentist's Hunch
As stated earlier, most dentists make a risk assessment for their patients during the first meeting. It has been demonstrated that this assessment can be a valid predictor of risk.

Risk Categories
Generally the practitioner is advised to categorise caries risk into either high, moderate or low.

In the view of the authors, the moderate category does not add any value and it is better to use the dichotomy of "requires extra prevention" or "no intervention beyond what the patient is already doing".

The Carious Process

In order to understand the problems associated with the diagnosis of dental caries, an understanding of the disease process is essential. This is also necessary if we are to adopt a modern biological and evidence-based approach to its prevention and management.

Coronal caries occurs on three sites:
- Free smooth surfaces
- Approximal surfaces
- Pits and fissures.

Although not the only theory postulated for the aetiology of dental caries, the acidogenic theory has overwhelming evidence to support it. Miller, in 1883, concluded that caries results from decalcification caused by bacterial acid production followed by bacterial invasion and the destruction of any remaining tissues. The causes for the initiation and progression of caries are multifactorial. Over a period of time, caries can occur on a susceptible tooth surface in the presence of cariogenic bacterial plaque and bacterial substrate.

Pits and fissures are predilection sites for caries because they are stagnation areas, inaccessible to cleaning and thus the removal of bacterial plaque. Occlusal surfaces benefit less than smooth surfaces from the caries preventive action of fluoride.

The crown of a tooth consists of (from the surface inwards) enamel, dentine and the dental pulpal tissues (pulp). The dentine and pulp are often considered to be a single complex. Enamel is the most highly mineralised tissue in the human body (92% by volume; 97% by weight). The degree of mineralisation of dentine, although high, is less than that of enamel (48% by volume; 69% by weight).

Pits and fissures generally occur:
• in the occlusal surface of the molars and premolars.
• the palatal surface of incisors, canines and molars.
• the buccal surface of lower molars.

The pathological features of caries in pits and fissures are similar to those seen in smooth surface caries but it is generally assumed that differences in surface form result in a later clinical (macroscopic) presentation.

Enamel Caries
In the mouth, the enamel surface is in a state of ionic flux. Below pH 5.5 mineral is eventually lost and this can lead to the formation of caries. At higher pH levels, and particularly in the presence of fluoride, this process is reversed.

White spot detection
The first visible sign of enamel caries, the white spot lesion, is relatively easily identified on free (exposed) smooth surfaces (Fig 2-3). However, it is often impossible to diagnose in pits and fissures because of surface morphology. White spot lesions are more obvious when teeth are dry. This is because of the different refractive indices of enamel, water and air. Sound enamel has a refractive index of 1.62. When demineralised, enamel becomes porous, if the teeth are wet the lesion has a refractive index approaching that of water (1.33) and will appear opaque compared to sound tissue. If dried, the water in the pores is replaced with air of refractive index 1.0 and the lesion becomes more obvious. To detect white spot lesions, teeth should be clean and dry

Microscopy of a white spot
In ground section the established white spot lesion can be described as hav-

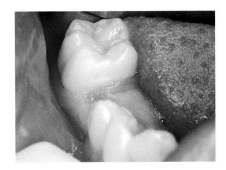

Fig 2-3 White spot.

ing four zones, the optical properties of which reflect differing degrees of mineralisation and lesion activity (Fig 2-4):

- **Zone 1** - The translucent zone is the first recognisable histological change at the advancing edge of the lesion.
- **Zone 2** - The dark zone is the second recognisable histological change. It is thought that the dark zone is narrow in rapidly advancing lesions and wider in more slowly advancing lesions when remineralisation is occurring.
- **Zone 3** - The body of the lesion is the third histological zone.

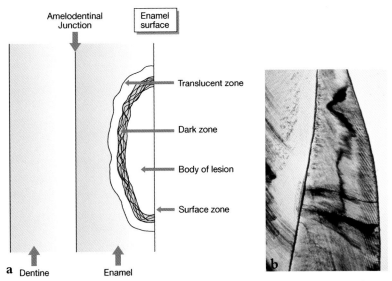

Fig 2-4 (a) The zones of an enamel carious lesion on a smooth surface. (b) Ground section of an enamel carious lesion in polarised light.

15

- **Zone 4** - The fourth histological zone is the surface zone. This zone is approximately 40μm in width. The surface of normal enamel differs in composition from the deeper layers; it is more highly mineralised and has, for example, a higher fluoride level and a lower magnesium level. It has been suggested that there may be areas of the enamel surface, which, because of their particular structure, are less resistant to acid attack than neighbouring areas. Thus, acid is allowed to penetrate into deeper layers in some of these areas, resulting in sub-surface demineralisation. However, if the enamel surface is cut away and an artificial caries is induced in the exposed surface the lesion still shows a relatively unaffected surface zone. A possible explanation for this relatively normal surface zone is that it represents an area of reprecipitation of mineral derived both from the plaque on the surface and from mineral dissolved in deeper regions of the lesion. In the surface and dark zones, the enamel crystals are of greater diameter than found in sound enamel. This is evidence of remineralisation in these areas.

Progression of Enamel Caries

The first stage in the carious process is surface demineralisation. This is followed by the development of a subsurface translucent zone, which is unrecognisable clinically and radiographically. Enlargement of the subsurface translucent zone leads to the development of a central dark zone. As the lesion enlarges more mineral is lost and the centre of the dark zone becomes the body of the lesion. At this point the caries is clinically recognisable as a white spot (Fig 2-3). The caries may then become stained by exogenous pigments derived from food and become clinically recognisable as a brown spot (Fig 2-5).

If the caries reaches the amelodentinal junction (ADJ) it spreads laterally and in this way the enamel may become undermined, giving a bluish-white

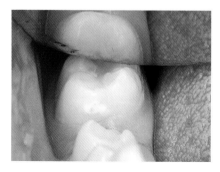

Fig 2-5 Brown spot.

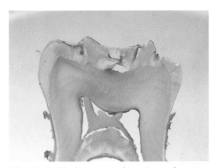

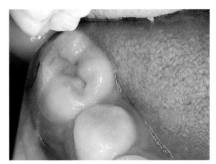

Fig 2-6 Caries extending into dentine and undermining the enamel.

Fig 2-7 The bluish-white appearance of undermined enamel.

appearance to the enamel clinically (Figs 2-6 and 2-7). This lateral spread may be related to the relatively high organic content and low fluoride content of this part of the enamel, although this concept of lateral spread has recently been questioned, and it has been suggested that the histological extent of the lesion on the surface is the same as its extent at the ADJ. Extension along the ADJ results in undermining of sound enamel adjacent to the lesion. The final stage is breakdown of the surface zone with formation of a cavity, although this stage may sometimes occur earlier in lesion formation — for example, while the lesion is still confined to enamel.

Enamel Caries in the Fissures
Fissure caries is frequently of multicentric origin, lesions developing independently and coalescing over time. As the enamel caries progresses, it extends towards the dentine "guided" by the orientation of the enamel prisms. At the base of the fissure it may coalesce with lesions present on the other surfaces of the fissure, forming a cone with its apex towards the enamel surface. The area of dentine initially involved, should the lesion progress, is therefore large compared with that of a smooth surface lesion. The lesion on a smooth surface is also a cone but with its apex towards the dentine surface.

Caries of the Dentine–Pulp Complex
Unlike enamel, both the dentine and the dental pulp are vital tissues. The two tissues are so intimately connected that they are best considered as a single complex. The odontoblast processes extend into dentine: dentine receives its blood supply from the pulp. This dentine-pulp complex is capable of reaction and repair to a stimulus such as caries (Fig 2-8a–b).

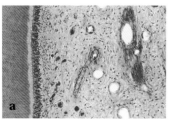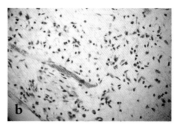

Fig 2-8 Dental pulp (a) healthy and (b) inflamed.

If the caries reaches the ADJ, the caries will spread laterally to involve a large area of dentine. Dentine demineralisation does not occur until the enamel lesion has reached the ADJ, although reactive dentine may form before this.

The histological zones found in dentine caries
As with the caries in enamel, the lesion in dentine has been described as having a number of zones (Fig 2-9):
- **Zone 1** – Sclerosis
- **Zone 2** – Demineralisation
- **Zone 3** - Bacterial invasion
- **Zone 4** – Destruction.

Some researchers describe only two layers (zones) in carious dentine:
- An ***outer layer*** of dentine, which is irreversibly denatured, infected, and cannot be remineralised (infected layer).
- An ***inner layer*** reversibly denatured but not infected (affected layer).

The concept of two layers of caries in dentine, the infected and the affected, is the key to modern caries management.

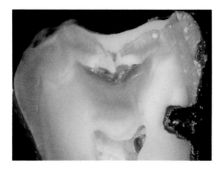

Fig 2-9 Zones of the caries in dentine can be thought of from a histological and biological viewpoint.

Caries progression through dentine

The rate of progression of caries through dentine is variable. In fact, progression is not inevitable — the caries can arrest. In rapidly progressing caries, the necrotic dentine is very soft and yellowish-white. In chronic or arrested caries, the dentine is hard and brownish-black in colour. If dentine caries does progress unchecked, it may lead to irreversible pulpitis and loss of vitality of the tooth.

Cariology in Primary Teeth

Caries are no different in primary teeth than in permanent teeth but there are some issues to be considered when primary and permanent teeth are compared (Fig 2-10).

Primary teeth

- are smaller
- the enamel is thinner
- the pulp is relatively larger
- the pulp horns are nearer to the surface
- there is more aprismatic enamel present in the enamel of primary teeth
- the contact points between posterior primary teeth are flatter and wider
- than permanent teeth.

The anatomy and morphology of primary teeth lead to more rapid progression of caries and make the clinical visual identification of demineralisation more difficult. Fortunately, the pulps of primary teeth have the same potential to heal or produce secondary dentine as their permanent counterparts.

Caries Diagnosis

Caries diagnosis is difficult. Even among well-trained and experienced clinicians there will be variation in detection, diagnosis and, for that matter, treatment-planning. A caries diagnostic examination should be broken down into a number of stages: detection, diagnosis, and recording (Fig 2-11). Clinicians all too frequently record what they see as a treatment decision rather

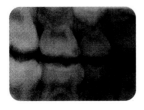

Fig 2-10 Bitewing radiograph illustrating the differences in morphology between permanent and primary teeth.

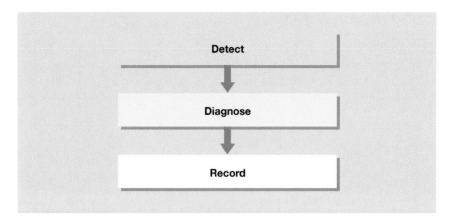

Fig 2-11 The caries diagnostic process.

than a diagnosis, for example, a mesial cavitated dentine lesion in a lower right first permanent molar recorded as "MO amalgam".

The Caries Diagnostic Examination

Clinical Visual
The clinical visual examination consisting of five stages forms the basis of caries diagnosis (Fig 2-12).

Systematic
Always start at the same place in the mouth — there is a logic in making this the most distal surface in the upper right quadrant and working clockwise to the lower right, as this ties in with the FDI tooth notation (Fig 2-13). For every tooth, work round its surfaces in a systematic manner, as it is all too easy to miss the lingual surfaces of lower teeth or the buccal surfaces of upper teeth (Fig 2-14).

Clean
Dental plaque is not translucent, so to diagnose even quite advanced lesions it must be removed (Fig 2-15). For some reason dentists have historically provided an examination followed by a polish. It is much more sensible for the patient prior to examination to brush their own teeth to remove the plaque. This also presents the opportunity to provide advice to the patients on toothbrushing ability. Polish the patients teeth prior to attempting to diagnose caries.

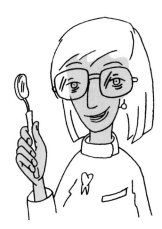

Fig 2-12 Visual inspection is the foundation of caries diagnosis.

Illumination

The dentist requires a light source to make diagnosis possible. In addition to good illumination provided by a suitably positioned operating light, the use of a light source will facilitate transillumination (Fig 2-16).

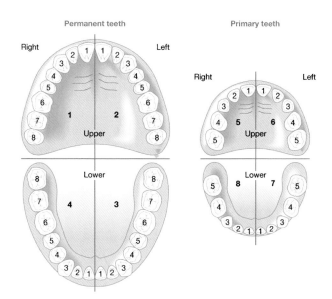

Fig 2-13 FDI notation: secondary and primary teeth.

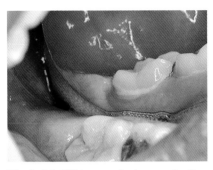

Fig 2-14 White spot lesion on the lingual surface of tooth 46, with the possibility of more advanced lesions on the mesial and distal surfaces. These can easily be missed.

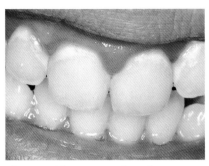

Fig 2-15 Plaque on surface of permanent incisors, making diagnosis of the caries present impossible.

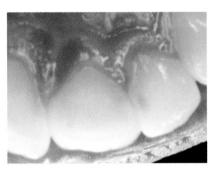

Fig 2-16 Transillumination of anterior teeth, demonstrating the dark shadow of the approximal lesion present on the mesial surface of tooth 12.

Dry

The detection of caries in its early stages relies on the differences in the porosity and therefore refractive index of carious versus sound dental hard tissue. When we dry the teeth we will have the ability to detect disease at its earliest visible stage (the white spot lesion). Classification systems have been developed that use the appearance of the teeth wet and dry to classify the stage and activity of the disease.

Drying the teeth helps with caries activity assessment:
- A white spot enamel lesion has a matt enamel (acid-etched appearance) surface; this frequently indicates an active lesion.
- A lesion with a glossy surface is often arrested.
- It is almost impossible to detect the subtle differences between matt and gloss without first drying the affected surface.

Put the sharp probe away!
For many years a visual-tactile examination rather than a purely visual examination was the mainstay of caries diagnosis. This should no longer be the case for a number of reasons:

- The use of a probe does not improve the accuracy of caries diagnosis.
- Probing of a demineralised site (which has the potential to remineralise) will further destroy the enamel structure creating an iatrogenic cavity and preventing any possibility of remineralisation.
- There is the possibility of inoculating other sites with cariogenic bacteria.

For these reasons, a sharp probe has no place in caries diagnosis (Fig 2-17). All that the diagnosis of a sticky fissure tells you is that there is a good fit between the probe and the fissure. However, a blunt probe, such as a periodontal probe, can be used to remove plaque from fissures using a dredging motion. As it can be problematic determining if a brown spot lesion is cavitated or not, the side of a blunt probe may also be used to confirm if a surface has broken down.

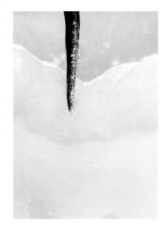

Radiographs
A visual clinical examination will detect only some of the enamel and dentine carious lesions that may be present. Therefore, it needs to be sup-

Fig 2-17 Probes do not improve the validity of occlusal caries diagnosis.

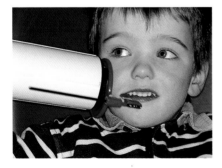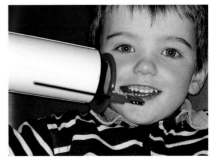

Fig 2-18 (a, b) With explanation and understanding it is possible to take bitewing radiographs of young children though they may initially be apprehensive.

plemented by radiological examination. The views that are of value for caries diagnosis are:
- bitewings
- orthopantomogram (OPT)
- bimolars
- periapicals.

Bitewings
Bitewings are the first choice view for caries diagnosis. Bitewings provide information on both occlusal dentine caries and approximal enamel and dentine caries (Fig 2-18a-b and Fig 2-10).

Orthopantomogram (OPT)
OPT is not the first choice for caries detection but when these are available they do provide useful information. OPT can detect the presence of an occlusal dentine carious lesion with a high degree of accuracy. Proximal surface lesions can also be seen on OPT but with much lower accuracy than with bitewings.

Bimolar view
Bimolars are not as useful a view as bitewings because there is often overlap of structures. However, they are of use in the pre-cooperative child who will not cope with bitewings or an OPT.

Periapicals
Periapicals are as accurate as bitewings for caries diagnosis, but obviously less information is available on any one film. The key role of the periapical view is in the diagnosis of periodontal disease and the diagnosis and monitoring of dental traumatic injuries.

Processing and viewing radiographs
It is important that the radiographic and processing techniques are of a high quality. Just as important are the viewing methods and conditions:
- a systematic approach
- viewing box
- blacked-out viewing box
- magnification.

How frequently should a radiographic examination be performed?
Bitewing radiographs should be considered for all children from the age of four years and above who are at risk of caries. However, not all children can

tolerate the placement of the film at this age. The clinician should ask the question "Why not take bitewings?" rather than "Why take bitewings?". Radiographs at an early stage will detect approximal enamel caries, thus offering the opportunity for the dental operator and patient (parent/carer) to take preventive action before the caries become more advanced and consequently more difficult to treat. The frequency of radiographic examination needs to be based on a thorough caries risk assessment. The dentist has to balance the benefits of the additional diagnostic yield with the risks of exposure to ionising radiation.

Adjuncts and Novel Aids to Caries Diagnosis

Magnification

Restorative dentists are increasingly using magnification to assist with the preparation of teeth. Magnification can also help with the detection and diagnosis of caries (Fig 2-19).

Fibre Optic Transillumination (FOTI)

FOTI helps with the detection of approximal enamel and dentinal lesions, and it can also be used to detect occlusal dentinal caries (Fig 2-20). In general, a 0.5mm tip is used for approximal lesions and a 5mm tip is used for occlusal surfaces. However, the smaller diameter tip is just as appropriate for occlusals as the operator just has to move it over the surface. Clinically, FOTI can be used

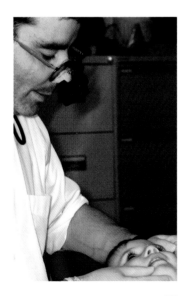

Fig 2-19 Magnification loops.

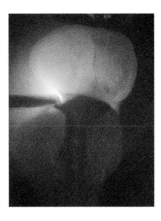

Fig 2-20 FOTI probe in the embrasure between the teeth. The shadow of a dentine carious lesion is visible.

in a number ways — for example, the dentist can use it routinely at every examination helping to decide if radiographs are indicated. It can also be used to provide further information when, despite a thorough clinical visual examination and radiographs, the clinician still remains unsure. One particular use of FOTI is to help differentiate between staining and caries on the occlusal surface.

Temporary Tooth Separation (TTS)
The placement of an orthodontic separator to move the teeth apart allows direct visual access to a surface for diagnosis. This approach has two significant advantages over bitewing radiography:
- The avoidance of exposure to ionising radiation.
- The ability to detect whether the surface is cavitated.

The process of separation takes about three to four days. The tooth returns to its original position following removal of the separator within hours. TTS can be used at specific individual sites or for all contacts, limiting radiographic exposure. This brings us to one of the drawbacks of TTS: the patient may experience some discomfort while the separator is in place, and this discomfort is likely to be greater if all contacts are separated (Fig 2.21a-d).

Laser Fluorescence
Laser florescence can be used to assist with the detection and diagnosis of caries. The currently available commercial device (Diagnodent, KaVo Germany) measures the fluorescence of the porphyrins made by bacteria in the caries. This device is designed for the diagnosis of occlusal caries but it can be used on accessible smooth surfaces. It is not designed to be a screening tool, where it is likely to generate a number of false positive diagnoses, but

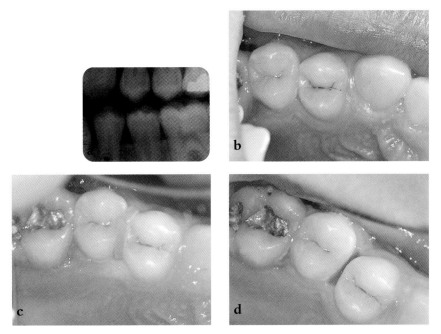

Fig 2-21 (a) Bitewing radiograph showing radiolucency 15 mesial and 14 distal. There are also lesions at 15 distal and 46 mesial. (b) The clinical appearance of teeth 14 and 15. (c) Separator in place between teeth 14 and 15. (d) Four days after removal of the separator the surfaces can be assessed directly. In this case both surfaces are intact and white spot enamel caries lesions are present.

to aid the dentist with equivocal lesions. In use, the dentist applies the probe tip to the tooth surface under investigation and a digital reading indicates the status of the surface through sound to deep dentine caries (Fig 2-22a-b).

Electric Caries Meter (ECM)

Enamel is a very poor conductor of electricity. However, following carious attack the enamel becomes more porous and the ions present in the pores in the lesion will conduct electricity with much less resistance than sound enamel. This is the principle behind the working of the ECM (ECM Lode Netherlands). Like the laser fluorescence devices, the ECM is principally of use on occlusal surfaces. All methods of caries diagnosis and detection rely on attention to detail but ECM is perhaps the most technique-sensitive. Of particular relevance to paediatric dentistry is that the ECM is not reliable on immature teeth, frequently indicating caries when it is not present (Figs 2-23).

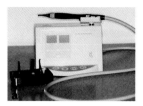

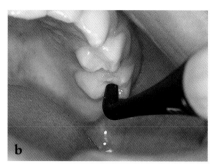

Fig 2-22 (a) Laser fluorescence devise (b) DIAG-NOdent probe on the occlusal of 85.

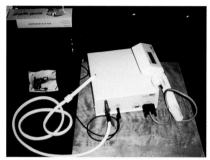

Fig 2-23 Electric caries meter.

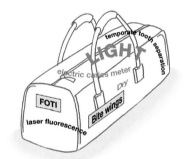

Fig 2-24 The caries diagnosis "Toolkit".

All of the above methods have both advantages and disadvantages, but they should be considered a toolkit from which the dentist selects to improve the accuracy of caries detection and diagnosis (Figs 2-24).

Recording Caries

Having completed a meticulous examination the clinician must record what has been found. This aids with treatment–planning and also allows the monitoring of lesion progression and regression at subsequent recalls.

A simple system for recording the finding of a visual examination, which is suitable to general dental practice and current charting methods, is given in Table 2-1.

All too often only dentine caries is recorded, disregarding valuable information. The clinician should attempt to record as much on all lesions detected as possible, no matter which diagnostic tool has been used.

Table 2-1 **Recording a clinical visual examination**

Code	Diagnosis
W	An active white spot enamel lesion.
WI	An inactive white spot enamel lesion.
B	An active brown spot enamel lesion.
BI	An inactive brown spot lesion.
D	Dentine caries.
DA	Arrested dentine caries.
P	Caries extending to the pulp.

A similar approach can be used for radiographs recording the extent of the lesion. A useful system was proposed by Pitts (1984), and an adaptation of Pitts system is given in Table 2-2.

Table 2-2 **Recording caries diagnostic information from radiographs**

Code	Diagnosis
0	Sound.
1	Radiolucency (enamel lesion) extending up to halfway through enamel.
2	Radiolucency (enamel lesion) extending beyond halfway through enamel but not beyond the ADJ.
3	Radiolucency (dentine lesion) extending up to halfway through dentine.
4	Radiolucency (dentine lesion) extending beyond halfway through dentine.
9	Excluded surface not readable.

Summary

- The dental, medical and social histories together with detailed knowledge of the child's diet, oral hygiene and fluoride usage are key components of caries risk assessment.
- The caries risk assessment should be recorded in the notes; this will assist in determining best practice, particularly the effective targeting of prevention and frequency of radiographs.

- Understanding caries progression in enamel and onwards into the dentine-pulp complex can assist in diagnosis.
- The anatomy and morphology of primary teeth lead to both caries reaching the pulp faster and making visual diagnosis more difficult.
- The stages of a caries diagnostic examination are:
  - detection
  - diagnosis
  - record- keeping.

Practical Tips

- For caries detection: Clean, Illuminate and Dry.
- Bitewing radiographs are the first choice view for caries diagnosis.
- Perform a caries risk assessment.

Further Reading and References

Ekstrand K, Ricketts DN, Kidd EA. Occlusal caries: pathology, diagnosis and logical management. Dental Update 2001;28:380-387.

Kidd EAM, Joyston-Bechal S. Essentials of Dental Caries. 2nd edition. Oxford: Oxford University Press, 1997.

Pitts NB. Systems for grading approximal carious lesions and overlaps diagnosed from bitewing radiographs. Proposals for future standardization. Comm Dent Oral Epidemiol 1984;12:114-122.

Scottish Intercollegiate Guidelines Network National Guideline 47. Preventing dental caries in high-risk children. Edinburgh: Royal College of Physicians, 2000.

Chapter 3
Treatment Planning and Managing Toothache

Aim

The aim of this chapter is to outline the principles of treatment planning. The management of the child with toothache will also be considered. The treatment of reversible and irreversible pulpitis will be compared and presented within the wider context of caries risk, the child's potential for cooperation and the degree of parental support.

Outcome

On completing this chapter, the practitioner should feel confident in treatment planning and in the management of toothache in children and in the selection of the appropriate method of achieving pain control.

Introduction

Although dental caries is almost completely preventable, some parts of the UK have amongst the highest prevalence of the disease in Western Europe. The number of carious teeth that are treated by restoration is low, and this is particularly the case when primary teeth are considered. Indeed, the demand for general anaesthesia for removal of carious teeth is by far the most common reason for an out-patient paediatric hospital admission in many regions of the UK. The reasons for this are complex and relate to socio-economic status, ethnicity and geographic location. The solutions are equally complex and many are beyond the scope of the individual practitioner and therefore beyond the scope of this text. But how can the dental team manage a child with toothache?

Pragmatic treatment planning

Correct diagnosis is only the first part in the formulation of the treatment plan. The final piece of the treatment plan jigsaw is determined by measuring the likely compliance of the child and the level of parental support and consent. The best treatment plans are pragmatic – in other words, they will only be successful if they are achievable in the first place.

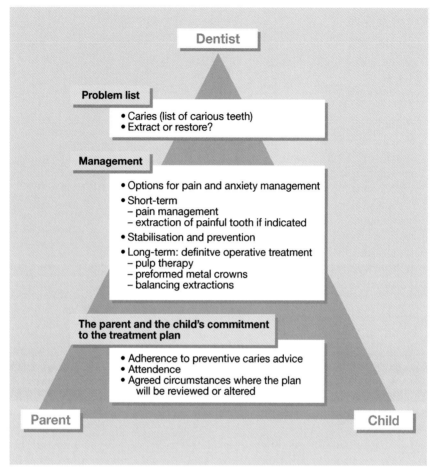

Fig 3-1 The conference between the dentist, child and parent is essential to success.

Dental treatment cannot be carried out without parental consent. This means that the parent or carer has a role in developing the definitive treatment plan. This is particularly true when the different treatment options (if there are any) are discussed. Therefore, the dentist has to explain the disease process to the patient and parent in a language they will understand. He/she also has to explain the management, and this is best achieved by demonstrating both the clinical and radiographic findings (Fig 3-1).

Problem List

A problem list can help focus the dentist's attention on the important factors that determine the shape of the treatment plan. These factors include pain, caries risk, cooperation and the potential complexity of the operative treatment options.

The Stages of a Treatment Plan

A treatment plan is made up of a number of stages:

- relief of pain
- prevention at home
- professional prevention
- stabilisation of caries present
- restorations
- pulp therapy
- extractions
- behaviour management
- reinforce prevention.

This system of planning care is based on putting prevention first after pain relief and is the focus of the treatment plan. Preventive treatments, particularly those provided by the patient and their family at home every day, will have the greatest long-term benefit on the patient's oral health. There is also a hierarchy of treatment, commencing with simple, pleasant procedures, moving on as the patient's confidence and compliance increases, to more technically demanding and perhaps more unpleasant ones.

Following extractions or other unpleasant procedures it is wise to end the course of treatment with a pleasant visit focusing on prevention. This will provide positive reinforcement and help erase unpleasant memories.

Analgesia, Sedation and General Anaesthesia

There is no doubt that restorations placed under local anaesthesia are superior in terms of quality and longevity. Unfortunately, not all children can cope with local anaesthetic injections at their initial presentation.

Depending on the child's age, cooperation and the nature of the planned procedure, there may be a need for a decision on the appropriateness of sedation (usually inhalation sedation) or general anaesthesia to help the child cope with the required operative care. The choice to use either sedation or, particularly,

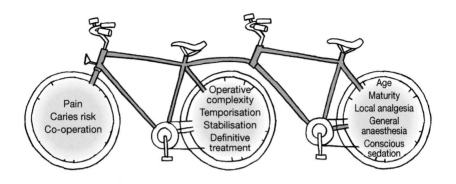

Fig 3-2 The final plan depends on the problem list and the expectation of how the child will cope to accept treatment.

general anaesthetia should always be made with a full assessment of the risks and benefits and consideration of any possible alternatives (Fig 3-2).

The Child with Toothache

Diagnosis of toothache relies on a thorough history and examination. Even though this chapter focuses on toothache, the dentist must take care to exclude other causes of pain.

Common causes of oral pain in children include:
- abscesses,
- caries (often no pain),
- trauma,
- tooth wear,
- infection,
- soft tissue lesions (i.e. recurrent oral ulceration),
- exfoliation/eruption.

Reversible or Irreversible Pulpitis?
The key to managing toothache, especially in primary teeth, is determining whether or not the pulpitis is reversible or irreversible. The correct diagnosis can be elicited through the history and the clinical and radiographic examination. A summary of this is shown in Table 3-1.

Table 3-1 **Differentiating between reversible and irreversible pulpitis in children**

	Reversible Pulpitis	**Irreversible Pulpitis/Abscess**
History	• Precipitated by sweet, hot, cold • Pain stops when stimuli are removed • Short duration • Mainly occurs when eating	• Constant • Relieved only by analgesics • Kept awake • Previous symptoms of reversible pulpitis but these were untreated and eventually ceased
Examination	• Absence of signs and symptoms of reversible pulpitis • Early carious lesion(s)	• Lymphadenopathy • Raised temperature • Extensive marginal ridge breakdown • Sinus • Intra-oral swelling
Radiographs (Bitewing radiographs produce the highest yield in caries detection)	• Caries into dentine	• Caries close to the pulp • Evidence of radiolucency

Caries Risk
The effective management of a child in pain has to pay due cognisance to their caries risk.

High caries risk
- Extraction might be more appropriate, especially if there are multiple carious teeth.
- The ideal plan should include the management of all the other carious teeth.
- A preventive regimen should be initiated following initial pain relief.

Low caries risk
- The caries extent and presence of pulpitis may indicate that extraction of the painful tooth is required.
- Consider whether balancing extractions are required.
- Other carious teeth might be restorable.
- The ideal plan should include the management of the other carious teeth.
- A preventive regimen should be initiated following initial pain relief.

Assessing Compliance
The potential compliance of the child depends on:
- The past dental history.
- The success of previous treatment (remember they may be more mature now).
- Their general demeanour (the child may be fractious due to toothache and sleep loss).
- Previous attendance pattern — regular attenders may be more familiar with the dental environment and more likely to accept treatment.

Restore or Extract?

The decision to keep the tooth depends on (see Fig 3-3):
- Diagnosis of reversible or irreversible pulpitis.
- Likelihood of pulpal involvement (i.e. the tooth will require a vital pulpotomy to successfully restore it).
- Quality and quantity of remaining tooth tissue.
- Previous extractions and edentulous spaces.

Reversible Pulpitis
Restore if possible but especially when:
- The majority of the other carious teeth are restorable.
- The child is compliant.
- The parent is keen to save the teeth.
- There is good reason to save this tooth (e.g. hypodontia or space-maintainance).

Extract when:
- Other carious teeth may need extraction and it may be wise to balance.
- The child is non-compliant.
- There is no parental support for restoration.
- The family is unlikely to attend beyond pain relief.

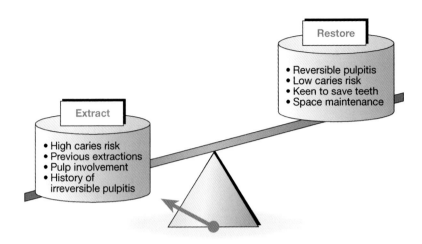

Fig 3-3 Restore or extract?

Irreversible Pulpitis or the Non-Vital Tooth

Try to restore if:
- The majority of the other carious teeth are restorable.
- The child is compliant.
- The parent is keen to save the teeth.
- There is no medical contraindication to pulp therapy.
- There is good reason to save this tooth (e.g. hypodontia or space-maintenance).

Extract when:
- Other carious teeth may need extraction and it may be wise to balance these.
- The child is non-compliant.
- There is no parental support for restoration.
- The family is unlikely to attend beyond pain relief.
- The tooth is not restorable.

Restore: Temporise

The placement of a temporary dressing (Fig 3-4) may be effective in relieving pain in teeth with reversible, irreversible pulpitis or even non-vital teeth. In the

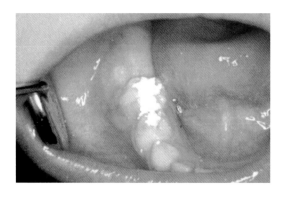

Fig 3-4 A temporary dressing can provide pain relief.

case of a tooth that is not scheduled for restoration, antibiotic/steroid paste may provide relief. In primary teeth, medication used for pulpotomy may also be used to provide temporary pain relief until extraction can be arranged. In the case of reversible pulpitis, where restoration is planned, the temporary restoration should be a material that is not detrimental to the health of the pulp and produces a good seal (e.g. glass ionomer or zinc oxide eugenol cement).

Balancing and Compensation?
- Balancing is the extraction of a tooth in the same arch.
- Compensating is an extraction in the opposing arch.

Balancing and compensation are indicated to maintain symmetry, in particular to avoid a centre-line shift of the permanent incisors, which may avoid the need for more complex orthodontic treatment later (Fig 3-5). The evidence supporting balancing and compensating extractions in the primary dentition is scant. However, most orthodontists and paediatric dentists would agree with the following, particularly in an individual without spacing:
- Always balance the extraction of primary canines.
- Do not balance the extraction of primary second molars.
- Compensatory extractions in the primary dentition are never indicated.
- The more crowded the dentition, the greater the need to balance.

Exceptions are:
- Where a primary molar or canine has already been lost from the contralateral side, resulting in a centre line shift and space closure, this requires a full orthodontic assessment.
- The spaced primary dentition — balancing is not indicated.

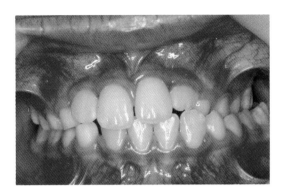

Fig 3-5 A centre-line shift.

First Permanent Molars

When extraction of the first permanent molars is necessary, the appropriate time to consider this is between the ages of nine to 10 years, when the bifurcation of the second permanent molar is starting to calcify. At this point, the mesial movement of the second permanent molar tooth is likely to close the space created by the extraction of the first permanent molar. If extractions are delayed until the roots of the second permanent molars are forming the potential for space closure is reduced. Earlier extraction, which is sometimes enforced, increases the risk of distal movement of the developing second premolar.

In general terms:
- These balancing and compensating extractions are usually enforced extractions due to caries and apply mainly to children with Class I occlusions.
- If the extraction of an upper first permanent molar is required then the lower tooth is treated on its own merits and retained, provided it is of good prognosis.
- When the extraction of a lower first permanent molar is indicated the opposing tooth should also be extracted. If this opposing tooth is not extracted there is a risk of it over-erupting and in the process preventing the mesial drift of the lower second permanent molar and therefore space closure.
- There are numerous exceptions to this rule, such as in Class II and Class III malocclusions and in cases of hypodontia. A specialist opinion is usually indicated before embarking on the extraction of first permanent molars in the developing dentition in these circumstances.

Analgesia and Antibiotics

Analgesics should be used to provide pain relief. In children the drugs of choice are paracetamol or ibuprofen. These should be prescribed according to the manufacturers' instructions.

Antibiotics do not reliably relieve the symptoms of pulpitis. Even in cases where pain relief is achieved there can be a delay of at least a day before any effects are felt. The inappropriate prescription of antibiotics leads to the growing problem of antimicrobial resistance. There is also a risk of an allergic reaction when any drug is prescribed. For these reasons, antibiotics should be reserved for the patient who has systemic symptoms, such as pyrexia, trismus or facial swelling.

The Benefit of Drainage

Whenever the child's cooperation will allow, drainage of an abscessed tooth is the treatment of choice. This gives almost immediate relief of symptoms and often prevents the need to prescribe antibiotics.

Drainage can be achieved either by accessing the pulp chamber, using rotary instruments, or by incision of the soft tissues. A pointing fluctuant intra-oral swelling can be incised with the aid of topical anaesthetic or ethyl chloride applied to a cotton wool roll. The incision of a swelling that is not pointing is frequently futile.

Drainage through the pulp chamber is best done following administration of local anaesthetic to avoid the danger of causing pain by accessing a tooth with remaining vital tissue. The local anaesthetic technique used should avoid injection into a region of infection. Where the practitioner is sure that no vital tissue remains this procedure can be performed without local anaesthetic. In such clinical cases, this is a quick and simple method of providing pain relief even in young children with little or no experience of dental care.

Where the tooth being drained is to be extracted it can be left open to drain, but not for a prolonged period. Where endodontic therapy is planned the tooth should be sealed as soon as possible. The only indication for leaving these teeth open for any extended period is when the pus is continuing to drain.

Managing the Child with Active Caries

The continued presence of bacterial plaque on the tooth surface both initiates and then continues to drive the carious process forward. If there was no plaque there would be no caries, no matter how advanced the lesion. Unfortunately, once cavitation has occurred it generally becomes impossible to remove plaque effectively. Therefore, under such circumstances stabilisation becomes the only appropriate option in the high caries risk child, slowing down caries progression while the definitive restorations are being undertaken and the preventive treatment provided.

Stabilisation
If the caries can be isolated from the plaque on the surface by the placement of a dressing following removal of caries at the margins of the lesion, caries progression will slow and possibly arrest. Even if it is not possible to remove any caries, a dressing may still buy time. In the case of occlusal lesions, without obvious cavitation, the placement of a pit and fissure sealant may slow or arrest lesion progression. In the case of an occlusal lesion with obvious cavitation it may be appropriate to place a glass ionomer dressing before sealing. This approach helps provide the support necessary for the relatively brittle sealant (Fig 3-6).

Stabilisation is of particular value for:
- The pre-cooperative patient — preventing lesion progression until definitive restoration is possible.
- The patient with multiple carious lesions — arresting caries progression over the course of a long treatment plan.
- The use of an indirect pulp cap or as part of serial excavation — avoiding the need for endodontic therapy.
- Prevention of sensitivity in teeth in proximity to the one being restored but outside the anaesthetised area.

The Sequence of Operative Care

Where possible, operative care is commenced in the maxillary buccal segments because this is where painless local analgesia is best achieved. Block injections should be delayed until the patient has grown in confidence and understanding. This confidence will follow after experiencing painless infiltration local anaesthesia.

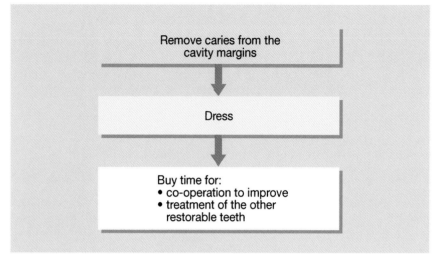

Fig 3-6 The sequence of stabilisation.

Operative care must be integrated with preventive therapy otherwise new lesions will develop in the caries-active child during the course of the operative treatment.

A typical operative sequence is as follows:
- **Step 1** – Temporary dressing (stabilisation)
- **Step 2** – Placement of fissure sealants
- **Step 3** – Simple (minimal) restorations where no local analgesia is required
- **Step 4** – Restorations, pulp therapy or primary molar extractions in the posterior maxilla with local analgesia
- **Step 5** – Operative treatment requiring a mandibular block (treat the whole quadrant)
- **Step 6** – Anterior restorations.

Practical Tips

- When explaining a treatment plan do not take any knowledge for granted.
- Present the "problem" list.
- Make the plan appropriate to the child's (and their parents') needs, desires and abilities.
- Put prevention first.

Further Reading

Chadwick BL, Hosey MT. Child Taming: How to Manage Children in Dental Practice. Quintessentials Dental Series Vol. 9. London: Quintessence Publishing Co. Ltd, 2003.

Chapter 4
The Caries Prevention Tool Kit and How to Use it

Aim

The aim of this chapter is to equip the dental team to successfully prevent caries in children. The reader will become familiarised briefly with community-based programmes so that these can be more easily identified locally to facilitate linkage between the community and general dental services. Following this, the focus will shift to how preventive care can be individualised and delivered to children and their parents within the dental surgery environment based on the prior assessment of caries risk.

Outcome

On completing this chapter the practitioner should be equipped with contemporary knowledge to provide preventive care for individual children and understand how community-based programmes might complement this effort.

Introduction

There is nothing more soul-destroying than carefully restoring a carious dentition for a child only to find new caries at a subsequent review. Children with carious primary teeth are at greater risk of developing caries in their permanent dentition. Ideally, we would hope that our child patients remain caries free in the first place. But how can this be achieved?

Contemporary research informs us that oral health education is best when delivered to infants. Hence, many community-based schemes are now focussed on nursery schools and linked to antenatal classes and health visitor contact with new mums. But how can the busy dental practice contribute towards this, and what can be done in the dental surgery to prevent caries in high-risk children?

It is already understood that caries is the result of the simultaneous long-term presence of oral commensals (most notably *Streptococcus mutans*), a car-

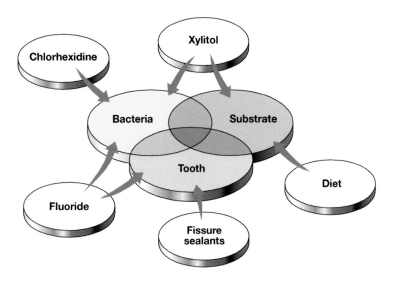

Fig 4-1 Caries aetiology and prevention tools.

bohydrate substrate and a susceptible tooth surface. Caries aetiology and prevention tools are shown in Fig 4-1.

The Caries Prevention Tool Kit

The cornerstones of caries prevention are:
- diet modification
- fluoride
- fissure sealants
- chewing gum (Xylitol)
- chlorhexidine.

Diet Modification
The cornerstone of diet counselling to prevent dental caries is to:
- reduce the amount of sugar consumed
- limit sugar frequency to meal times only.

For diet modification to be effective it must be:
- personal

- pertinent
- positive.

Avoid making parents feel guilty
Parents genuinely wish to avoid dental caries developing in their children, so in the event of caries development they can feel guilt. Remember, the selection of less cariogenic food is difficult:
- Sugar content is not always clear in food-labelling.
- Access to healthy foods can be difficult in socially deprived areas.
- Healthy foods can be a more expensive option in socially deprived areas.
- Not everyone can cook.
- The sugar industry spends more on marketing and advertising (just watch Saturday morning children's TV) than the government has to spend on the provision of dental health services for children.
- Few families stick to the "three square meals a day" epithet and favour a grazing/snacking style.
- The child may be looked after in a nursery school, by a child minder or by another relative during the day.
- School tuck shops are tempting.

Personalised advice using a diet diary
- A three-day diet diary can help the dental team and the parent work together to highlight sugar consumption and then to reduce the amount and frequency of cariogenic foods.
- The instructions for use are:
  - use for three consecutive days
  - give the times and amount, and food brand if possible
  - one of the days should include a Saturday or Sunday.

When reviewing the diet diary:
- Ask the patient or parent (carer) to identify where they feel the problems are.
- Offer alternative non-cariogenic foods.
- Recommend alternatives that will fit in with the family life-style.
- Remember to preserve the child's dignity in front of their peers (e.g. a trendy water container to facilitate the transition from sugared pop to water).

Remember, many diet diaries are not accurate because:
- The patient is worried about being reprimanded.
- The patient wants to please you, so gives you what they think you want to see.
- Be particularly suspicious of diaries written with the same pen.

Non-milk extrinsic sugars
Parents are often confused by food labelling of sugars. Even the best-educated and best-intentioned families can unwittingly consume an otherwise "healthy" diet that has a high sugar content — drinks labelled "no added sugar" being a common trap and culprit.

Foods that cause caries:
• sweets
• biscuits and cakes
• drinks and juices.

Popular misconceptions (foods that DO cause caries):
• plain biscuits
• some flavours of crisps (e.g. prawn cocktail flavour)
• sauces and salad dressings
• yoghurts
• dried fruits
• "low sugar" drinks
• "no sugar added" drinks
• soya milk
• breast milk if continued beyond normal weaning time
• access to juice or milk through the night.

Alternative snacks:
• crackers
• bread
• bread sticks
• carrot sticks
• slices/pieces of fruit (children may not feel able to eat a whole fruit but may eat a slice)
• hard cheese.

Fluoride

The benefit of fluoride in caries prevention has been known for half a century. Many cities in the USA have fluoridated water supplies, and other parts of the world have natural fluoridated water. In the UK, parts of Northumbria and the West Midlands have been fluoridated for over 30 years.

How does Fluoride Prevent Caries?

Fluoride acts both systemically and topically. Its anti-caries effect can be summarised as follows:

- alters the ameloblast
- makes fissures more shallow
- stabilises the matrix of the hydroxyapatite molecule within enamel, making it more resistant to acid dissolution
- interferes with glycolysis, slowing down bacterial acid production
- has direct anti-bacterial effect
- its principal anti–caries action is to alter the balance of remineralisation v. demineralisation in favour of remineralisation.

Fluoride gives greatest protection to smooth surfaces

Prescribing Fluoride

The simple rule of thumb to prescribing fluoride is:

- select only ONE systemic method
- select ANY NUMBER of topical methods (Table 4-1).

Table 4-1 **Systemic vs. topical fluoride prescribing**

Systemic Fluoride	Topical Fluoride
Water	Toothpaste
Tablets	Varnish
	Mouth rinse

Fluoride Toothpaste

Caries rates have been falling gradually around the world over the past few decades. This fall can be almost solely attributed to the introduction of fluoride toothpaste. Indeed, toothpaste is bettered only by water fluoridation as the most effective method of delivering the preventive benefit of fluoride.

When asking a patient to brush more frequently or teaching them to brush more effectively, we are reinforcing practice of an already social norm. Therefore, this is often an easier behaviour modification to achieve than dietary change.

As well as toothbrushing being an effective method of delivering fluoride, when performed properly it reduces the build-up of plaque, thus helping to eliminate one of the aetiological causes of caries. It has been suggested that one of the reasons the occlusal surface of erupting molars are particularly caries-prone is that plaque builds up on these surfaces and is not removed by mastication because the teeth are not in occlusion. The emptive process can take over a year. This problem is compounded by the difficulty in effectively brushing these teeth.

Fluoride Dose and Caries Reduction
The magnitude of the caries reduction is entirely dependent on the dose of the fluoride (Table 4-2):
- the higher the dose of fluoride in toothpaste, the greater the reduction in caries
- children at high caries risk should have at least 1000ppm fluoride in toothpaste
- spit out after brushing but don't rinse with water.

Table 4-2 **How much fluoride is in toothpaste?** (Adapted from: Creasey SJ. Fluoride in Toothpaste. Br Dental J 1994;176:330.

Brand	Fluoride Level (ppm)
Boots Children Gel	163
Punch & Judy	1053
Mentadent	1461
Signal	1500
Colgate 0-6	395
Boots Tom & Jerry	526
Tesco Bubble Gum	526
Super Drug Strawberry Gel	1053

Swallowing and Eating Toothpaste

Unfortunately, few infants can spit out toothpaste after brushing and some children like the taste of it so much that they eat it. Therefore, despite the link between dose and efficacy in caries reduction, some care in prescribing is required. Even the size of the toothbrush head surface can be a determinant of the amount of toothpaste used, so:

- only use a pea-sized amount of toothpaste
- select a small-sized toothbrush for children
- suggest that the toothpaste is applied across the bristles rather than lengthwise
- parents must supervise children toothbrushing until they are at least seven years old.

Caries Risk Assessment and Fluoride Dose

The dose of fluoride toothpaste to prescribe depends on the caries risk of the child.

- a child with a low caries risk = up to 600ppm fluoride
- a child with a high caries risk = 1000ppm fluoride.

The risk of fluorosis to the incisors is negligible in children aged over six years and they can safely start to use the adult strength toothpaste (1500ppm).

Fluoride Varnish

The topical application of a fluoride varnish is a method of delivering a very high fluoride dose (1mL contains 22.6mg of fluoride) to the smooth surfaces most susceptible to caries. Almost all of the fluoride in the varnish will eventually be ingested, so take care not to overdose. The varnish adheres to a dry surface best, therefore the tooth should be dried whenever possible. Flossing fluoride varnish through contact points also increases its effectiveness (Fig 4-2). There is a possibility of allergic reaction, especially with children with asthma.

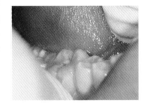

Fig 4-2 Floss fluoride varnish through the interproximal contacts with care.

Fluoride Tablets

Fluoride tablets act systemically and topically if they are sucked before swallowing. The original dosage was based on the assumption that a child would drink at least one litre of water a day. This volume of consumption was later found to be too high and so the amended fluoride tablet dosages shown in Table 4-3 were implemented in 1997.

51

Table 4-3 **Fluoride supplement revised dosages**

Age	Tablet Dose (mg)
6 months - 3 years	0.25
3 - 6 years	0.5
> 6 years	1.0

Fluoride Mouthwash
To prescribe this:
- Daily rinsing is best with 0.05% fluoride.
- Use at a different time to toothbrushing so that salivary fluoride levels can be maintained throughout the day. Therefore, suggest a regime of brushing morning and night and use the mouthwash on returning home from school.
- The child needs to be capable of spitting out the mouthwash and thus they normally need to be over eight years of age.
- Use an alcohol-free variety (some mouthwashes have alcohol levels as high as 20%). Rinsing with alcohol has an adverse effect on the oral mucosa, and there have been reports of acute alcohol poisoning in children who have drunk mouthwash.
- All high-risk children and adolescents should be advised to use this approach but especially those with approximal caries.

Mottling
Approximately 10% of the population have a greater susceptibility to the effect of fluoride on their ameloblasts.

Management of enamel mottling
In its milder forms this is not necessarily unaesthetic but can be treated simply using the method of controlled enamel removal by acid–pumice micro abrasion (sometimes more correctly termed "abrosion") techniques. More severe mottling can be treated in adolescence by the provision of direct composite veneers followed by porcelain veneers in adulthood.

The Fluoride Future
New *in-vitro* research is suggesting that sustained, low-dose fluoride exposure may be the most efficacious means of reducing caries. Therefore, recent innovations such as the "fluoride bead" – a slow-release device, akin to tooth jewellery, may be of particular benefit in high caries risk children.

The Diagnosis and Management of Acute Fluoride Overdose
As little as 1mg/kg can cause toxicity. Symptoms include:
* nausea and vomiting
* stomach pain
* diarrhoea
* hypersalivation.

Overdose of 5mg/kg could be fatal. Symptoms include:
* convulsions
* respiratory and cardiac failure
* coma.

> *In 1000ppm toothpaste there is 1mg of fluoride in 1g.*

To manage overdose:
* Find out if any other poisons have been consumed.
* Give milk as a chelating agent (although the evidence for this is unclear).
* Establish dose (sometimes the dose can be unreliable since it is based on the communication between the dentist and the overwrought parent and so it is wisest to err on the side of caution (Tables 4-4 and 4-5).
* If in any doubt, send to hospital.

Table 4-4 **Overdose management is dependent on amount of fluoride ingested**

Dose	Action
Under 5mg/kg	Give milk.
5-15mg/kg	Give an emetic (Ipecac syrup): • 10mL for under 18 months old • 15mL for older children.
> 15mg/kg	Admit urgently to a paediatric intensive care unit.

Table 4-5 **Average child weights in relation to age**

Age	Weight
2 years	10kg
5 years	20kg
10 years	40kg

Fissure Sealants

Fissure sealants are a key component of the prevention tool kit in high caries risk children. Sealants should be applied to caries-susceptible teeth as soon as they erupt. Fissure sealants are technique-sensitive, and excellent moisture control is essential. Moreover, even after they have been carefully applied, fissure sealants require continued monitoring and will need replacing, should they begin to show signs of failure.

The teeth to fissure seal are:
- first permanent molars — occlusal surfaces and sometimes buccal pits
- palatal pits of upper permanent lateral incisors
- second permanent molars and all premolars.

Monitoring Following Placement

Failed fissure sealants do not cause dental caries, but if they become inadequate they cease to prevent it. Therefore, sealants should be checked at each recall. This includes:
- visual inspection
- check adequacy with a probe
- replace if defects are found
- use bitewing radiographs to monitor fissures where fissure sealants were applied over stains or fissure caries, particularly in high-risk children.

Which Fissure Sealant do I Use?

Unfilled (clear) fissure sealants

Unfilled fissure sealants can come in either clear or opaque. The opaquer is added colour rather than added filler. Unfilled fissure sealants are better than filled fissure sealants because:
- the material wets the surface better so it flows into the fissure more efficiently
- the material is easier to apply.

Filled fissure sealants
The theoretical advantage of improved wear resistance is balanced by their poorer ability to wet the surface. This means they flow and penetrate the fissure less well. The poorer wear resistance of the unfilled material is not a concern if the sealant flows well enough into the fissure.

To Light-cure or Not?
While there is perhaps little clinical difference between light-cured or self-cured fissure sealants in theory, light-cured materials set towards the light source. Therefore, they can be pulled away from the tooth surface forming shorter resin tags. In spite of this, dentists increasingly show a preference towards materials with a command set and so self-cured fissure sealants are becoming less readily available.

Sealing Over Caries
A well-applied fissure sealant can arrest dentinal caries but the mechanical properties of the material determines that this may be a short-term rather than a long-term solution, particularly if there is cavitation. As such, it is a method of stabilising caries progression in an anxious child when coupled with continued preventive care and behavioural management.

Enamel Biopsy
When do you open up the fissure? This decision is dependent on the appearance of the caries on bitewing radiographs.
• If the enamel is stained (suggestive of enamel caries) but there is no dentine caries on the bitewing radiographs, seal over the stain and monitor the adequacy of the fissure sealant.
• Laser fluorescence or electric caries meter devices may have a role in helping with this decision.
• If the caries extends minimally into dentine the restoration of choice is a preventive resin restoration.
• If in doubt following radiography — seal and monitor.

Xylitol Chewing Gum

Xylitol is a type of sugar but it can reduce dental caries because it is not fermentable by oral commensals and inhibits *Streptoccocus mutans*. Indeed, when it is an ingredient of chewing gum, salivary flow is stimulated to give additional caries reduction.

In Swedish studies, the caries prevalence in six-year-old children, whose mothers were given Xylitol gum to chew during and after pregnancy, was less compared to controls. In this way, the maternal load of *Streptococcus mutans* was reduced, and so less was transmitted to the newborn child.

- Some children might readily consider Xylitol chewing gum to be an acceptable alternative to sweets and mints.
- There are side-effects of the use of sugar substitutes, such as Xylitol, in the gastrointestinal tract, resulting in increased flatulence and diarrhoea.
- There may also be safety concerns regarding the use of artificial sweeteners in young children.
- Suggest the use of Xylitol gum to expectant mothers who are at high caries risk.

Chlorhexidine Varnish

The anti-bacterial agent chlorhexidine is also available as a varnish. This may have some benefit in high caries risk adolescents. However, the evidence to support its use is not conclusive and so fluoride varnish would still appear to be the better choice. Chlorhexidine and fluoride varnish should not be applied at the same visit, as they both function by adhering to the tooth.

Community-Based Programmes

The delivery of health education in the community focuses on:
- nursery schools
- breakfast clubs, where children are encouraged to start the day with a healthy meal
- antenatal classes and health visitors.

The dietary habits of a lifetime are established early in life, even before birth. The help of health visitors and antenatal classes in educating expectant mothers is valuable. Children who are at high caries risk often develop caries in their primary dentition before they start school. By the time a child reaches adolescence their lifestyle is set and more difficult to modify. Breakfast clubs help to ensure that a child is less hungry mid-morning and so less likely to snack. They also inspire healthy eating practices, and the small fee charged commits pocket money that might otherwise be spent in the "tuck shop".

The New Dental Team

The new-extended dental team for the oral health care of children now includes:
- dental hygienist
- dental health educator
- dental therapist.

Multi-Disciplinary Teams

It is not just dentists and professionals complementary to dentistry (PCDs) who can be enrolled to help deliver dental preventive education and to promote dental health. Doctors, professions allied to medicine and schoolteachers can all play a part in the campaign for better oral health for our children. In some parts of the UK, these are grouped into "oral health action teams" (OHAT) or "oral health cooperatives" – a focussed grouping of individual professionals with the aim of primary medical and dental care within a given region or area.

Table 4-6 **A prevention plan for a high caries risk child living in a non-fluoridated area (less than 0.3ppm)**

Prevention "Tool"	How to...	Frequency
Diet	• Three-day diet diary • Personalised advice • Positive messages • Monitor and encourage	• At initial visit then monitor at subsequent reviews
Fluoride★	• Topical varnish • Fluoride toothpaste 1000ppm • Supplement (tablet or mouthwash dependent on age)	• Twice yearly • Twice daily • Daily
Fissure sealants	• Fissures and pits (permanent molars and lateral incisors)	• On eruption
Xylitol gum	• To expectant mums • Adolescents	• Each visit
Chlorhexidine	• Interproximally	• Three-monthly

★ Children in fluoridated area do not need a fluoride supplement.

Table 4-7 **A prevention plan for a low caries risk child**

Prevention "Tool"	How to...	Frequency
Diet	• Personalised advice • Positive messages • Monitor and encourage	• At initial visit then monitor at subsequent reviews
Fluoride	• Varnish • Fluoride toothpaste 600ppm until age 4-6 years	• Erupting molars • Twice daily
Fissure sealants	• Consider only if fissures are stained	
Xylitol gum	• Only if risk level changes	
Chlorhexidine	• Only if risk level changes	

Personalising Preventive Care

In Tables 4-6 and 4-7 a risk-dependent schematic of preventive treatment is presented. It is worth noting, however:
- This approach does not replace the dental operator's own judgement as she/he strives to give each child patient individual care.
- It is essential to continually monitor each child and ensure that their medical/dental history is updated.
- A child's caries risk can change with time (e.g. going to a new school with free access to a "tuck shop" or taking up a new or possibly more strenuous sport, resulting in the frequent consumption of glucose-containing drinks).

Practical Tips

- Prescribe only one systemic but as many topical vehicles for fluoride.
- Spit, don't rinse after toothbrushing.

Further Reading

British Society of Paediatric Dentistry. Policy document on fluoride supplements and fluoride toothpastes for children. Int J Paediatric Dent 1996;6:132-142.

Murray JJ, Nunn JH, S teele JG. Prevention of Oral Diseases. 4th Edition. Oxford: Oxford University Press.

Scottish Intercollegiate Guidelines Network National Guideline Number 47. Preventing Dental Caries In High Risk Children. Edinburgh: Royal College of Physicians, 2000.

Chapter 5
Intracoronal Restorations for Posterior Primary Teeth

Aims

The aim of this chapter is to discuss the intracoronal restoration of carious primary teeth. In addition, the clinical relevance of the anatomical differences between the primary and permanent dentitions are highlighted.

Outcome

After reading this chapter, the practitioner should feel able to perform modern operative approaches to caries removal and intracoronal restoration of primary molar teeth and understand how these relate to the morphology of primary molars.

Introduction

Parents and dentists alike are keen to avoid the spectre of toothache in a child. Primary teeth have a key role to play in the future development of both occlusal development and in the acceptance of the child by their peers. The anatomical form of primary teeth, especially primary molars, means that caries can cause changes in the pulp faster than in permanent teeth. Fortunately the restorative techniques are simpler compared to permanent teeth and profit from primary tooth morphology.

Anatomy

The anatomical differences between primary and permanent teeth are illustrated in Fig 5-1. Compared to a permanent tooth, the anatomy of a primary tooth can be summarised as follows:

- The enamel is thin, lighter in colour and easier to cut with a bur compared with enamel of permanent teeth.
- The crown is bulbous, especially towards the cervical area.
- There is a marked cervical constriction apical to the cervical bulge.
- In molars, the occlusal table is narrow in a buccolingual direction.
- The pulp horns extend high into the anatomical crown.
- The enamel rods are inclined occlusally in the cervical region.

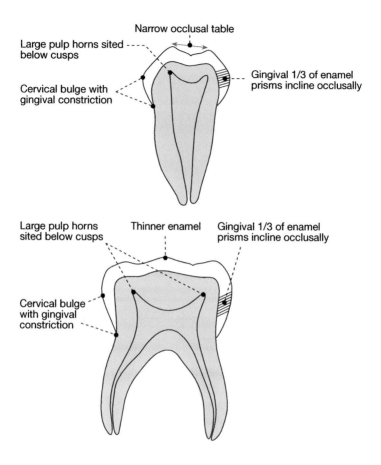

Fig 5-1 The anatomy of primary teeth.

Although the principles of caries removal in primary teeth are essentially the same as those for the permanent dentition, there are some differences that are important clinically. These are summarised in Table 5-1.

Table 5-1 **Clinical significance of primary toth anatomy**

Crown Morphology	Clinical Significance
Thinner enamel	• Short distances for caries to penetrate • Small burs used • Pulp horns near the enamel surface
Cervical bulge with gingival constriction	• Tendency to make floor of box too deep • Forced to re-establish floor by moving axial wall towards pulp
Narrow occlusal table	• Cusps can be weakened by over-extending buccolingual dimensions
Broad contact areas located gingivally	• Buccal and lingual walls of a box need to clear contact especially near floor of the box
Large pulp horns sited below cusps	• Isthmus must be narrow to avoid pulp exposure • To reduce failure of restorative material, pulpoaxial line angle may be deepened to increase bulk of material
Gingival third of enamel prisms incline occlusally	• No need to bevel cavosurface as enamel rods on floor of box will be supported

Indications for Restoration

A minimal restoration, placed with relative ease when the lesion has just penetrated dentine and cavitated, can avoid the need for a larger restoration or even extraction later. In this way, dental operative procedures can be kept simple and used in combination with preventive care to ensure a positive attitude to dentistry and life-long oral health.

Primary teeth are restored in order to:
• Prevent pain and sequelae, such as irreversible pulpitis and infection.
• Avoid extraction in certain medical conditions (e.g. bleeding disorders).
• Avoid extractions in anxious children.

- Preserve masticatory function.
- Maintain an intact arch (primary dentition).
- Provide space maintenance (mixed dentition).
- Maintain anterior aesthetics.

Sequential Planning

For most children, a period of acclimatisation is required before embarking upon a restorative approach. Remember to use language that is appropriate to the age of the child. In the very young, access for caries removal can be improved by the use of miniature burs in a miniature handpiece. If a child has experienced caries in the primary dentition, you should consider fissure sealing the first permanent molars upon eruption.

Cavity Preparation

In general, the same principles and approach apply to the preparation of primary teeth as for the permanent dentition, but there are several factors worthy of consideration when treating dental caries in primary teeth: moisture control, the longevity of restorative materials, the extent of the caries in relation to the pulp horns and the cooperation of the child.

Moisture Control

Ideally, this should be achieved using dental dam isolation, but lack of cooperation may lead to compromise. Good moisture control can be achieved using small saliva ejectors, cotton wool rolls and dry guards (Fig 5-2).

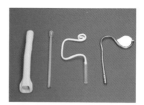 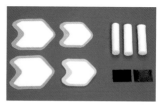

Fig 5-2 Equipment used to obtain moisture control (a) suction and saliva ejectors. (b) Cotton wool rolls and dry guards.

Choice of Material and Durability of Restorations

When placing a restoration in a primary tooth the dentist has to decide whether the filling is to last the lifetime of the tooth or if it is a temporary restoration that she/he expects to eventually replace. This choice is dependent on various factors, not least the expected longevity of the tooth. Nevertheless, in terms of durability the selection of materials can be summarised as follows:

- Plastic restorations, such as amalgam, composite resins and glass ionomer cements perform best in one or two surface restorations. The glass ionomer materials have the advantage of directly adhering to tooth structure. They also release fluoride, although the clinical significance of this is unproven.
- The newer resin-modified glass ionomer cements and compomers have the advantage of directly adhering to tooth tissue and a command set due to the resin component. This may be helpful when dealing with a wriggly child.
- The more recent resin-modified glass ionomers and viscous glass ionomers have the advantages of glass ionomer but with improved strength.
- The compomers appear to have survival rates similar to amalgam in class II cavities and have the advantage of adhering to tooth tissue via bonding agents.
- The recommended restoration for primary molars with two or more carious surfaces is the preformed metal crown (stainless steel crown), and these restorations outperform other materials in all but the smallest of single surface restorations.

> *Two main factors affect the choice of material – those relating to the tooth to be restored and factors pertinent to the patient.*

Tooth factors
- The extent of the carious lesion (linked with durability).
- The cavity shape after caries removal (e.g. method of retention, maintaining healthy tooth tissue).

Patient factors
- Efficacy of isolation and moisture control (moisture-sensitive techniques).
- Caries rate (temporise initially to obtain caries control).
- Aesthetic expectations.

Caries in Primary Posterior Teeth

These can be put into the following subcategories:
- Pit and fissure caries.
- Approximal caries with pit and fissure caries.
- Approximal caries without pit and fissure caries.

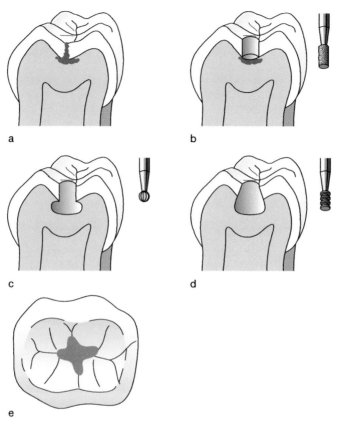

Fig 5-3 Occlusal pit and fissure caries removal. (a) Occlusal caries into dentine. (b) Access through carious enamel to carious dentine via straight diamond or steel flat fissure bur. (c) Caries removal leaving unsupported enamel, which should be removed. (d) Outline of cavity with a flat, slightly concave floor and walls diverging from the occlusal to provide retention for amalgam. (e) Outline is smooth without sharp angles and extends to include carious tissue only.

Useful Instruments for Caries Removal
- Small sharp excavators.
- Slow speed: round and flat fissure steel burs.
- High speed: small round and straight diamond burs.

Pit and Fissure Caries
Occlusal pit and fissure caries removal is shown in Fig 5-3.

Access
- Penetrate the occlusal surface within the carious area just into dentine (to a depth of 1.5mm x 0.5mm into dentine).
- A straight diamond high-speed bur may be used if the child can tolerate this. If not, use a steel flat fissure bur in the slow handpiece or slow speed diamond.

Outline
- Using a flat fissure or round steel bur, remove caries in pits and fissures, retaining oblique ridges wherever possible.
- Aim for a flat, slightly concave floor.
- If amalgam is to be used, the walls must diverge from the occlusal to provide retention.

Caries removal
- Remove remaining caries.
- Slow round steel bur or excavator.
- Clean walls, then floor, using gentle forces.
- Any undermined enamel should be removed to sound dentine.
- Aim for a smooth occlusal outline form without sharp angles.

Restoration
- If the cavity is deep or if an indirect pulp cap is indicated line the floor of the cavity using a hard setting calcium hydroxide.
- If amalgam or composite resin is used, a glass ionomer lining material may be used as an alternative to calcium hydroxide.
- In shallow and medium cavities no lining is indicated.
- Amalgam, compomer or glass ionomer cement may be used to restore the crown. If amalgam is used there must be sufficient mechanical retention within the cavity.
- Amalgam will tolerate some moisture contamination.
- Glass ionomer cement may be used as an alternative to amalgam similarly; compomer or composite if the child can cooperate with the use of a bonding system. "All-in-one" adhesive systems may simplify the bonding procedure enough to allow placement of compomer in some children.
- If a large area of occlusal table is to be restored, consider placing of a preformed metal crown.

Approximal Posterior Lesion without Pit and Fissure Caries (Retentive Box)
Often with this type of lesion there is no cavitation occlusally (see Fig 5-4).

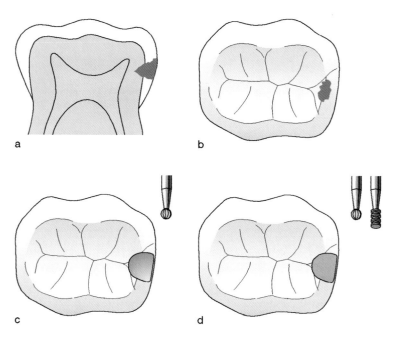

Fig 5-4 Approximal caries removal without pit and fissure caries. (a-b) Approximal lesion involving dentine, without pit and fissure caries. (c) Access gained at carious marginal ridge using a round steel bur, extending to remove caries at buccal/lingual/palatal walls. A sliver of enamel between cavity and adjacent tooth remains. (d) Remove sliver of enamel with a fissure bur and ensure floor of box is just beyond the contact area. The cavity outline may be wide at the base of the box because of the need to clear the wide contact area.

Access
Access is still obtained from the occlusal surface, but the preparation has no occlusal extension or key:
- Penetrate the enamel immediately inside the marginal ridge.
- Once through enamel, the bur will "drop" into the carious dentine.

Caries removal
Gaining access will leave a sliver of enamel between the cavity and adjacent tooth.

Buccal and lingual walls
- Extend the buccal and lingual/palatal walls to remove caries and gain access to caries at the amelodential junction and the dentine beyond.

- Clearing the broad contact area may produce a wide cavity outline.
- Small round and fissure steel burs can be used.

Floor
- Remove carious dentine using slowly rotating steel burs.
- The floor of the box should be just beyond the contact area with an occlusal slope to follow enamel rod orientation.
- Do not over-deepen the floor as this will lead to pulpal exposure and "loss" of the floor due to the marked cervical constriction in primary molars.
- Remove the sliver of enamel with a slowly rotating fissure bur (or hand instrument) and smooth enamel margins.

Axial wall
- This should be just into dentine and parallel to the convexity of the tooth.
- If amalgam is to be placed, the buccal and lingual walls of the box must diverge from the occlusal to provide retention (this is also of value with adhesive materials). This may be supplemented by placing small grooves on the lingual/palatal wall and gingival floor using a 1/2 round steel bur.
- Care must be taken not to groove the buccal wall due to the proximity of the pulp horn.

Restoration
- A hard- setting calcium hydroxide or glass ionomer lining may be placed on the axial wall in deep cavities.
- A matrix band must be placed and if a tooth-coloured restoration is to be placed then the internal aspect of a metallic matrix strip should be smeared with a thin layer of petroleum jelly to prevent adherence to the metal.
- The material of choice to restore a retentive box is a compomer with an adhesive system.
- If amalgam is used, additional retentive measures must be taken as described previously.

Approximal Posterior Caries with Pit and Fissure Caries (Class II)
Access
It is best to produce the box part of the cavity first so that a decision on occlusal extension may be made with the help of some direct vision (Fig 5-5).

Box preparation
This is outlined in the previous section (retentive box), but grooves are not required within the box because an occlusal key will provide retention. If amal-

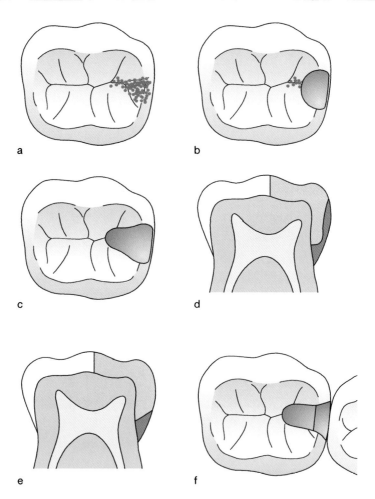

Fig 5-5 Approximal caries with pit and fissure caries removal. (a) Approximal, pit and fissure caries in a second primary molar. (b) Box preparation produced as for a retentive box (Fig 5-4) without grooves. (c) Isthmus width is 1/3 of width between buccal/lingual/palatal) cusps. Caries removal continued occlusally. (d) The floor of the box is sloping to follow the orientation of the enamel prisms. (e) The pulpo-axial line angle may be deepened centrally for extra bulk of material if amalgam is to be used. (f) The buccal/lingual/palatal walls of the box must clear the broad contact area with the adjacent tooth.

gam is to be used to restore this type of cavity, it will be at its thinnest in cross-section directly over the pulpo-axial line angle. To increase the strength of amalgam in this area (the isthmus), the line angle may be deepened by 1mm.

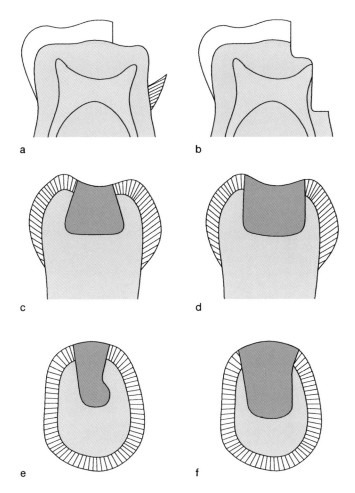

Fig 5-6 The correct and incorrect approaches to cavity design in the primary dentition. (a–b) Excess deepening at the floor of the box causes removal of dentine adjacent to the pulp horn resulting in pulp exposure. (c–f) An isthmus width of >1/3 of the width between buccal/lingual/palatal cusps will weaken cusps and increase the risk of pulp exposure.

Isthmus

- The isthmus width should be approximately 1/3 of the width between the buccal and lingual/palatal cusps.
- A wide isthmus will weaken cusps and increase the risk of pulp exposure (Fig 5-6).

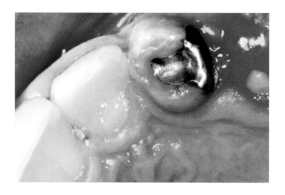

Fig 5-7 An amalgam restoration of approximal caries with pit and fissure caries in a maxillary first primary molar.

Pit and fissure caries
- Continuing from the isthmus, caries is removed and cavity outline established as described for pit and fissure caries.

Restoration
- A hard-setting calcium hydroxide or glass ionomer lining may be placed at the occlusal floor and/or axial wall of the box in deep cavities.
- Amalgam is still the material of choice, although its use is declining, but requires relatively destructive retentive features (Fig 5-7).
- Compomers may be used with an adhesive to conserve tooth tissue.

Practical Tips

- If the restoration is large, place a preformed metal crown (Fig 5-8).
- Miniature heads and miniature burs are useful in small mouths.
- Allow a child to have a rest and close the mouth during treatment that does not require stringent moisture control. They are then more likely to keep their mouth open when it is needed most.
- If, when using a glass ionomer cement, moisture control is difficult, place a square of thin green wax over the restoration to help keep it dry (Fig 5-9); alternatives to this are petroleum jelly or fluoride varnish.
- Fig 5-10 gives an example of a tooth-coloured restoration.

The Atraumatic Restorative Treatment (ART)

This technique was introduced in the early 1990s for use in developing countries. The ethos behind its development was to provide a combination of restorative and preventive treatment for primary and permanent teeth in areas of the

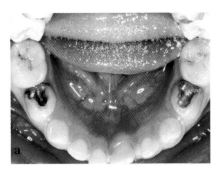

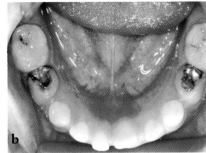

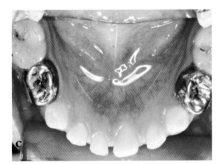

Fig 5-8 Amalgam restorations at (a) one year and (b) two years post-placement. (c) The teeth were subsequently restored with preformed metal crowns.

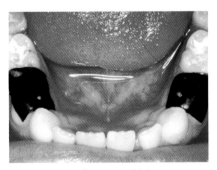

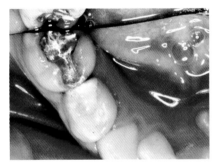

Fig 5-9 A small square of thin green wax placed over a setting glass-ionomer cement to prevent moisture contamination.

Fig 5-10 A tooth-coloured restoration of approximal and pit and fissure caries in a mandibular primary molar.

world where dentistry was inaccessible. A minimum amount of instruments and materials are required. Cole and Welbury (2000) have provided an excellent review of this technique, together with its possible uses in everyday situations.

Caries removal is undertaken using hand instruments only. It has been found by those experienced in this technique that local anaesthesia is rarely required. The cavity is then slightly overfilled with specially developed "condensable" glass-ionomer cement and a finger used to condense the material and force it into the pits and fissures remaining on the occlusal surface. This technique of condensation is known as the "finger-press" technique and aims to restore the cavity and seal the pits and fissures.

> *Studies have shown that one-surface ART restorations are the most durable. It can take up to 20 minutes to remove caries using hand instrumentation.*

ART has a possible role in the treatment of:
- dental-phobic patients
- part of an acclimatisation process in a young child
- mentally and physically impaired patients
- elderly patients.

ART Technique
Instruments
- tweezers
- excavators
- probe
- chisels/hatchets
- flat plastic/carver.

Access
- Isolate the tooth with cotton wool rolls.
- Clean tooth with water and cotton wool pledgets.
- Widen entrance to the carious lesion with hatchets.

Caries removal
- Remove all carious tissues using hand excavators.
- Clean with water and dry with cotton wool.

Restoration
- Consider pulp protection with hard-setting calcium hydroxide cement.
- Condition cavity walls (according to manufacturer's instructions).
- Place glass-ionomer cement into tooth, slightly overfilling the cavity.
- Apply pressure with a gloved finger over the occlusal surface.

- Remove excess material, with a carver or flat plastic, leaving pits and fissures sealed with glass-ionomer cement.
- Check the occlusion.
- Apply glass-ionomer varnish or petroleum jelly over the whole surface of glass-ionomer.

Practical Tips

- ART can be used as part of an acclimatisation process in the very young or anxious child.
- Single-surface restorations are more successful than multi-surface restorations.
- It is reported that caries removal may take up to 20 minutes with ART, so it is a good idea to plan for this beforehand.

Minimum Tooth Destruction

> *To remove dental caries, the aim is to prepare a cavity with minimum "invasion" of tooth tissue and with little or no discomfort for the patient.*

Conventional approaches to caries removal still involve the use of dental handpieces — high-speed to gain access and to establish cavity outline, then slow-speed to remove carious dentine. Many patients, particularly children, perceive the use of "the drill" as unpleasant.

With the advent of effective dentine-bonding agents and minimally invasive techniques such as the preventive resin restoration, we are able to be minimally invasive for small lesions. Added to this, we have seen the introduction of the technique of ART, air abrasion and the use of lasers for caries removal.

The Chemo-Mechanical Removal of Caries

The chemo-mechanical removal of carious dentine has been a concept that has existed for quite some time. However, the initial substance developed for "chemical" caries removal required the application of large volumes of gel to carious dentine to achieve its aim. It was considered unworkable to most operators and was not used widely. Technology in this area has moved forward, and products are now available which are useful, particularly for children who refuse to accept "the drill".

There are commercial kits available (e.g. Carisolv™). They contain two gels, which are mixed together to provide the active agent that separates carious from sound dentine. An advantage of modern chemo-mechanical cavity preparation is that sound dentine is not removed by the technique.

The active ingredients of the gel when mixed are:
- sodium hypochlorite (NaOCl)
- the amino acids glutamic acid, leucine and lysine.

The gel may also contain:
- methylcellulose (to increase viscosity of the gel, to improve handling)
- erythrosine (a dye so the gel can be seen easily).

The mode of action of this gel is:
- NaOCl is proteolytic and degrades organic substance at room temperature.
- Chlorine degrades denatured collagen, resulting in dissolution of the collagen fibre structure.
- The amino acids then attach to the protein chains of the carious dentine.
- The amino acids also prevent the degradation of healthy dentine by the hypochlorite.

The action of the gel results in separation of carious dentine from sound dentine.

The action of the gel can be improved by using specially developed hand instruments that have a scraping action rather than a sharp cutting profile (like excavators or burs). This is said to reduce the risk of removing sound dentine.

Chemo-Mechanical Caries Removal Technique
The manufacturers of these products claim that local anaesthesia is rarely required.

Instruments
- Two separate gels to be mixed together just before use. One contains hypochlorite and the other amino acids.
- The specifically designed non-cutting hand instruments.
- Cotton wool pledgets

Access
If the carious lesion has not cavitated, access to the carious dentine is required. This may well involve the use of a handpiece and bur.

Caries removal
- Cover the dentine caries with the gel.
- Wait 20 seconds for the gel to contact the dentine.
- Gently scrape the carious dentine with the hand instruments to remove softened dentine. When instrumenting, a light pressure should be used and different actions are employed depending on the specific instrument being used (e.g. whisking or rotating motion with the star-shaped instrument).
- The gel will become cloudy.
- Remove the gel by gentle washing or a cotton wool pledget and apply fresh gel to the dentine.
- Repeat the procedure until the gel remains transparent and the surface feels hard.
- Finally remove the remains of gel by washing gently with water or with a cotton wool pledget soaked in warm water.
- Dry the cavity with cotton wool.

Restoration
- Restore the tooth using an adhesive restoration.

Practical Tips For Chemo–Mechanical Caries Removal

- The activated gel has a short working life and should be discarded after approximately 30 minutes.
- This technique should only be used with the specially designed hand instruments.
- Cavity preparation, as with ART, is prolonged compared to more conventional methods. It may take up to 15 mins of gel applications and instrumentation to remove all carious dentine. The manufacturers have introduced a slow handpiece to decrease instrumentation times, but for a child who refuses to accept the handpiece this is of no benefit.
- Some children complain about the taste and smell of the gel, so good isolation is a positive benefit.
- If dentine caries is very near the pulp horn, then a carious exposure may occur following removal of carious dentine. If this outcome is suspected before treating the tooth, adequate pain control must be used, indirect pulp cap or a devitalising pulpotomy undertaken.

Lasers
Lasers do not have a significant role in the management of caries in the young child, in part because their use is intimidating. Secondly, they are of use only where direct line of sight access is possible.

Air Abrasion

This may have a role in the management of caries in the young child but remains unproven at present. One concern is the small particle size used, which makes the use of rubber dam mandatory.

Ozone

As with air abrasion the role of this technique in primary teeth remains unproven.

Further Reading

Cole BOI, Welbury RR. The Atraumatic Restorative Treatment (ART) Technique: Does it have a place in everyday practice? Dental Update 2000;27:118-123.

Ericson D, Zimmerman M, Raber H et al. Clinical evaluation of efficacy and safety of a new method for chemo-mechanical removal of caries. Caries Research 1999;33:171-177.

Fayle SA, Welbury RR, Roberts JF. BSPD. A policy document on the management of caries in the primary dentition. Int J Paediatric Dent 2001;11:153-157.

Chapter 6
Preformed Crowns Are Easy

Aim

To present the preparation and fitting of preformed crowns using a step-by-step approach to explain the technique.

Outcome

On completion of this chapter the practitioner should feel confident to use preformed crowns — so confident, in fact, as to dare to place them without a full trial fit.

Introduction

Many studies have shown that preformed crowns last significantly longer than other restorative materials used to restore caries in primary molars. However, relatively few are used despite the simplicity of the technique and the speed at which they can be placed. The reason for this under-use must be a perception that the technique is difficult or time-consuming. The crowning of primary molars using preformed crowns (Fig 6-1) is by no means similar to the provision of bespoke crowns for permanent teeth. In fact, some operators use a minimal preparation technique, simple trial fit and a basic kit.

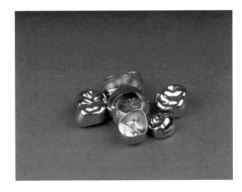

Fig 6-1 Preformed metal crowns for primary molars.

> *The key to the technique is to avoid cutting a shoulder.*

How are Preformed Metal Crowns Retained?

A primary molar tooth has a bulbous crown, much more so than a permanent molar tooth. It is this difference in tooth morphology that provides the retention of the crown as it slides over the bulbosity of the crown, to be held by the cervical constriction. Therefore, the preformed crown technique does not rely on either crown taper or crown height. This is the reason why a preformed crown can be used to restore even a grossly carious primary molar.

- A shoulder will prevent the crown from seating fully.
- Contouring the edge of the crown to fit snugly into the cervical constriction, a process known a "crimping", ensures a tighter fit.

Indications for Preformed Crowns for Primary Molars

- Large class II cavities.
- Badly broken down teeth.
- Following pulpotomy.
- Hard tissue anomaly (e.g. amelogenesis imperfecta or dentinogenesis imperfecta).

Instruments

- A fine-tapered diamond fissure bur as pointed as possible so that you can avoid cutting a shoulder (SHOFU PN ISO 0848 013, Fig 6-2) works well.
- An orthodontic band pusher (Fig 6-3).
- 114 Contouring "crimping" pliers (Fig 6-4).
- An orthodontic band remover (Fig 6-5).

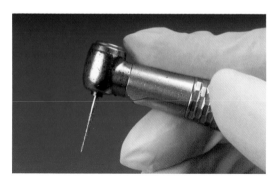

Fig 6-2 A fine-tapered diamond bur.

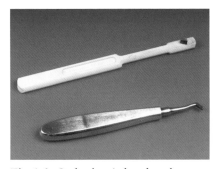

Fig 6-3 Orthodontic band pusher.

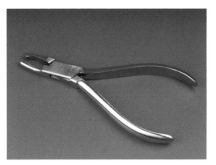

Fig 6-4 114 Contouring (crimping) pliers.

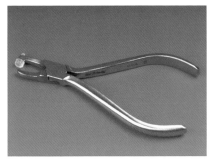

Fig 6-5 Orthodontic band remover.

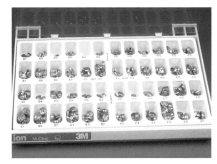

Fig 6-6 Preformed metal crown box.

Selection of the Crown

The crowns are marked with an indication of their size and position (Fig 6-6). There are two methods of choosing the best crown:

- Measure the mesiodistal width of the crown of the tooth in the mouth, or the available space with a divider, and then select the crown using this measurement.
- Trial and error (start with a size 4).

Step-by-Step Preparation and Fitting

This can be summarised as follows:
- Remove the caries.
- Prepare the tooth: "**O**cclusal: **A**pproximal: **P**eripheral".

- Select the crown:
    - try it in by placing it into the mesial and distal approximal areas
    - don't seat it fully - just check that it will "squeeze" down over the crown
    - remove it.
- Re-contour the crown margin, if this has been damaged, by using the crimping pliers.
- Cement the crown.
- Remove the excess cement.
- Check the occlusion.

Step One: Occlusal Reduction
- Reduce the occlusal height by 1.5 to 2mm.

Step Two: Approximal Reduction
- Use the tapered fissured bur for the proximal reduction.
- Place the bur on the mesial and distal marginal ridges and reduce the proximal surfaces.
- Start on the occlusal portion of the marginal ridge and sweep back and forth with bur moving cervically, until the interproximal gingivae can be clearly visualised.
- Produce a knife-edge finishing line (Fig 6-7).
- Check for ledges with an explorer and reduce even the slightest ledge since the crown will be prevented from seating (Fig 6-8).
- Performed crowns are made to fit properly only when both mesial and distal reductions are made.

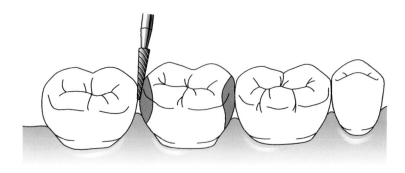

Fig 6-7 Mesial and distal reduction to produce a knife-edge finish.

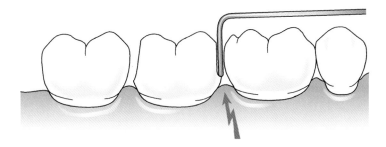

Fig 6-8 Check for a ledge since this will prevent the crown from fully seating.

Step Three: Peripheral Reduction
- Create a bevel between the occlusal table and the buccal, lingual and aproximal surfaces (about 1mm).
- Round off the sharp line angles, especially in the proximal areas (Fig 6-9).

Step Four: Try in the Crown
- Place the crown on the prepared tooth, using your finger or an orthodontic band seater.
- Then check the following:
    - mesial and distal contact areas (see if crown is wide enough)
    - occlusal - gingival height
    - buccal and lingual extension (see if crown is too wide)
    - occlusion.
- If the crown is fully seated, remove it using orthodontic band removers (Fig 6-10).

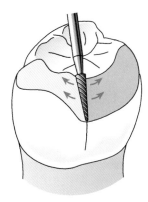

Fig 6-9 Peripheral reduction.

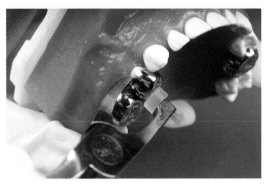

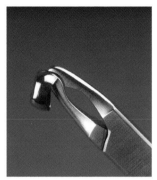

Fig 6-10 Using orthodontic band removers.

Fig 6-11 Use crimpers to correct the crown margin.

The correctly fitting crown seats with a snap: the operator can hear a click clearly as the crown snaps into place, but with growing confidence the operator will learn to judge the likely fit without fully seating it at this trial stage.

Step Five: The Gingival Contour

- Restore the crown contour at the gingival margin if this has been damaged during removal or if the crown failed to fit with a "snap" (Fig 6-11).

Step Six: Cementation

- Dry the crown.
- Isolate the tooth with cotton rolls.
- Dry the tooth.
- Place a creamy mix of glass–ionomer luting cement in the crown.
- Place the crown on the dry tooth and push to place with finger pressure or an orthodontic band seater.
- Remove cotton rolls and invite the child to bite.
- Remove excess cement interproximally using knotted dental floss before the glass- ionomer is fully set and buccal and lingually using a dental probe (Fig 6-12).

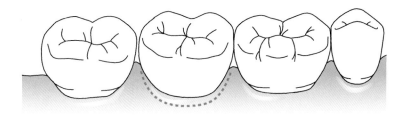

Fig 6-12 Crown in place. Note cervical extension of 1mm below the gingival margin.

Problem-Solving

Rocking
- If the preformed crown rocks this crown is either overextended or too wide (Fig 6-13).

Canting to One Side
- If the crown cants to one side as it is seated, uneven reduction of the occlusal surface may be the problem.
- Correct this by rounding the occlusal line angles.

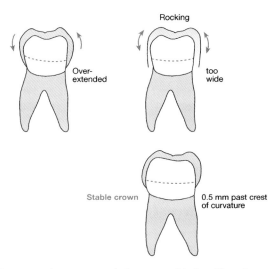

Fig 6-13 If the crown is overextended or too wide it will rock.

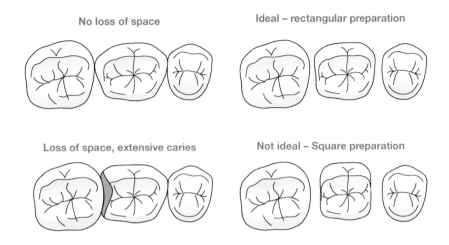

No loss of space

Ideal – rectangular preparation

Loss of space, extensive caries

Not ideal – Square preparation

Fig 6-14 Space loss in the lower arch.

Loss of Space due to Extensive Caries

Where caries has reduced the mesiodistal dimension of a tooth, resulting in space loss, fitting a steel crown can be difficult.

- *Upper primary molars are "square"-shaped*
- *Lower primary molars are "rectangular"-shaped*

Loss of Space in the Lower Arch

Ideally the prepared tooth should be generally rectangular in outline. When space loss occurs this outline becomes squarer in shape (Fig 6-14). The solution is to use the upper contralateral crown.

Loss of Space in the Upper Arch

The upper arch preparations are already square in shape but become more foreshortened due to caries. The solution is to reduce the tooth in a buccolingual direction to restore the square outline form needed for an upper preformed crown.

The Placement of Preformed Crowns with Minimal Preparation

In some instances it is possible to place preformed crowns with little or no preparation of the tooth, by having the patients bite to push the crown into place.

Work Steps for Placing Preformed Crown without Prior Preparation of the Tooth

- Explain the procedure to the patient.
- Remove any caries present using hand and rotary instruments (Fig 6-15).
- Select a crown — this is done using trial and error (start with a size 4). The crown should fit so that it feels that it will slip over the contact point. **DO NOT** place the crown at this point as it will be impossible to remove.
- Dry the tooth. Fill the crown with glass-ionomer cement and place on the tooth. As with a prepared tooth rotate the crown into place from the lingual surface. Press down into place with gentle pressure.
- Once the crown is vertically in place a cotton wool roll between it and the opposing tooth, then ask the child to bite down (Fig 6-16).
- An orthodontic band seater may help direct the force of the child's bite (Fig 6-17).
- Remove the excess cement.
- There may be some blanching of the gingiva. This is transient and not a cause for concern (Figs 6-18 and 6-19).

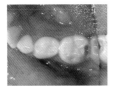 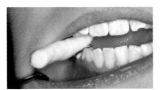 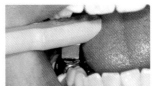

Fig 6-15 Tooth 85 after the removal of caries.

Fig 6-16 Child biting crown into place.

Fig 6-17 Child biting on orthodontic band seater to assist with placement of the SS Crown.

In many cases, because there has been no reduction in the occlusal height of the tooth, the preformed crown will be high. Due to dento-alveolar compensation the occlusal will readjust over the succeeding days. Pain does not

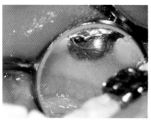

Fig 6-18 Do not be concerned by blanching of the gingival, this is transient.

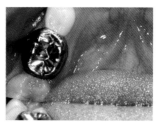

Fig 6-19 The crown in place.

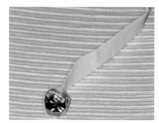

Fig 6-20 SS crown with autoclave tape attached to act as a "parachute chain" to protect the airway.

occur as a result of this, although the patient should be reassured that the temporary alteration in their bite is normal and will not last.

Advantages of the Minimal Preparation Technique
- Unless significant caries removal is required, local anaesthetic may be avoided.
- Relatively rapid atraumatic technique, of particular value in the anxious patient.
- Conservative of tooth tissue, a particular advantage with hypoplastic permanent molars.

A Practical Tip to Avoid Aspiration
It can be difficult to control and hold a preformed crown. If you are concerned that the crown my slip and endanger the airway or be swallowed, a strip of folded autoclave tape or elastoplast can be used as a handle (parachute chain). This is easily removed after the cement has set (Fig 6-20).

Practical Tips

- "**O**cclusal: **A**pproximal: **P**eripheral".
- Do not cut a shoulder.
- Use the upper contralateral crown to restore a lower molar that has suffered due to space loss.
- Use some knotted floss to clear cement from the contract points.
- Don't worry about initial gingival blanching — this will settle if the crown margin is well enough adapted.
- Use autoclave tape or elstoplast as a "handle" to avoid aspiration.

Chapter 7

Pulp Therapy in the Primary Dentition

Aim

The aim of this chapter is to demonstrate the simple pulp therapy techniques that are available to treat carious primary teeth. The rationale for their use will be discussed and each clinical stage demonstrated using a step-by-step approach.

Outcome

After reading this chapter the practitioner should be confident in performing the commonly used pulp therapy techniques for primary teeth.

Introduction

Why is there such an air of mystery surrounding primary molar pulp therapy in the UK? It is one of the most straightforward and quick procedures in the dental armamentarium. It involves simple medicaments and instrumentation and benefits the child two-fold: by avoiding the trauma of extraction and by preserving the space-maintenance role of the primary dentition.

Pulp therapy for cariously exposed primary molars aims to conserve the damaged tooth and restore its function until the permanent successor erupts. Successful treatment of pulp tissue reduces the need for unplanned extractions and the undesirable consequences that may follow.

In order to understand the principles behind the currently advocated pulp therapy techniques, the response of the pulp to a carious insult shall be discussed briefly. A simple step-by-step guide to the techniques will follow this. A complete list of the instruments and medication used is available at the end of this chapter. There have been recent changes to the medicaments available for pulp therapy in primary teeth. Confirmation by the International Agency for Research on Cancer (IARC) of the carcinogenic effects of formaldehyde in humans was published in June 2004. As a result, pulp therapy techniques are undergoing a period of significant change. This chapter is representative of the trend towards the use of aldehyde-free pulp therapy techniques in the UK.

Infected and Inflamed Dental Pulp

There are several reasons for a dental pulp to become inflamed or infected, but by far the commonest is as a sequel to dental caries.

Dental caries in a primary tooth progresses rapidly though the relatively thin enamel and penetrates dentine. The insult from bacterial toxins stimulates the underlying pulp to respond by mounting an inflammatory reaction (reversible pulpitis).

If a carious exposure occurs, microbes invade the pulp tissue, causing a massive increase in pulpal response. This is characterised by irreversible inflammation and tissue necrosis directly adjacent to the site of the exposure. If this remains untreated, bacteria and their products will progress through the pulp tissue, resulting in irreversible inflammation and tissue breakdown involving the whole pulp system. The spread of inflammation is gradual and progressive through the whole pulp and then beyond into the periradicular tissues via furcational, lateral and apical communications. The response of pulpal and periodontal tissues to such injury can lead to one of several outcomes:

- The periradicular tissues may become affected (periradicular periodontitis), with eventual involvement of associated soft tissue (Fig 7-1).
- If the exposure site involves a large area, hyperplastic pulpitis (pulp polyp) may occur (Fig 7-2).
- The tooth may be subject to pathological resorption — for example, internal inflammatory resorption (Fig 7-3).

If vital inflamed tissue is removed, leaving residual healthy pulp, it has the capacity to remain healthy if managed correctly. Therefore, the overall success of pulp therapy in the primary dentition depends upon:

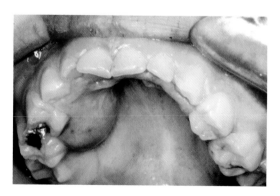

Fig 7-1 A palatal abscess associated with a grossly carious primary molar.

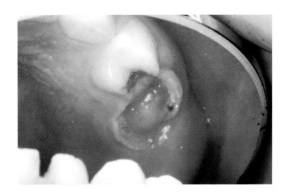

Fig 7-2 Hyperplastic pulpitis (pulp polyp) seen in the pulp of a primary molar.

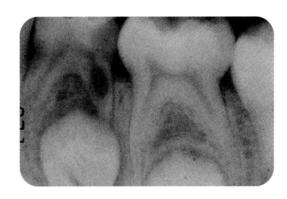

Fig 7-3 Internal inflammatory resorption affecting the distal root of a primary molar.

- Effective control of infection.
- Removal of irreversibly inflamed tissue.
- Appropriate wound dressing.
- Effective coronal seal during and after treatment.

When is Pulp Therapy Required?

- An accurate pain history is helpful in deciding the probable stage of pulpal involvement, but it is often difficult to obtain such information from a child.
- Preoperative radiographs are helpful to assess the extent of the carious lesion and its proximity to the pulp. They are also important to determine if periradicular pathology is present. Findings from radiographs can guide treatment decisions.

- Clinically, pulpal involvement can often be assessed more easily following caries removal. In other words, after caries removal look very carefully for evidence of pulpal exposure. Blood will be present at the exposure site if the pulp tissue is still vital coronally.
- If a carious exposure is bloodless, then some, if not all of the pulp, is likely to be necrotic.

Assessing Inflammation in a Vital Pulp

It can be difficult to assess the amount and level of inflammation within the pulp. Therefore, in vital pulp therapy it is assumed that the whole coronal pulp is "affected" and so all of the coronal pulp is amputated.

Following amputation of the coronal pulp, our attention must turn to the remaining radicular pulp stumps. The nature of the bleeding from the radicular pulp is used to assess whether inflammation has extended beyond the coronal pulp tissue and into the root canals. If haemostasis cannot be achieved, this tissue is assumed to be irreversibly inflamed and vital pulpotomy techniques are contraindicated. A tooth with persistent bleeding from the pulp stumps should be treated by pulpectomy.

Below are examples of signs and symptoms that could indicate that some form of pulp therapy is needed.

Signs

- Occlusal caries extending more than 4mm in depth.
- Approximal caries where 2/3 of the marginal ridge has been destroyed (Fig 7-4).
- Caries involving or very close to the pulp horns on a radiograph (Fig 7-5).

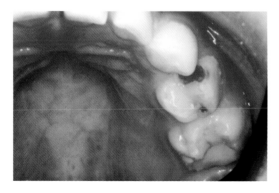

Fig 7-4 A primary molar with more than 2/3 of the marginal ridge broken down. This gives a strong indication that pulp therapy is required.

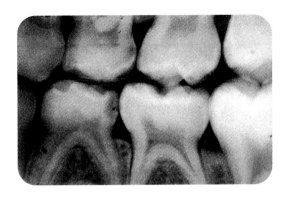

Fig 7-5 A radiographic view showing the proximity of an approximal carious lesion to the pulp.

- Mobility or tenderness to percussion.
- Sinus formation.
- Periradicular bone radiolucency on a radiograph.

Symptoms
- Pain
    - transient on thermal stimuli (reversible pulpitis)
    - spontaneous and lasting in nature (irreversible pulpitis)
    - from biting on the affected tooth (periapical or intraradicular infection).

Indications and Contraindications for Primary Molar Pulp Therapy

Further to the signs and symptoms, additional indications for pulp therapy are:
- Cooperative child and carers.
- Avoidance of the psychological trauma of extraction.
- Medical conditions where extraction should be avoided (e.g. haemophilia).
- Absence of the permanent successor tooth.
- To maintain an intact arch in the primary dentition.
- Space maintenance in the mixed dentition.

There are also several important contraindications to pulp therapy, including:
- Lack of cooperation from child or carer.
- Medically compromised children at risk from a dental bacteraemia (e.g. immunocompromised or at risk of developing infective endocarditis).
- Poor general condition of the mouth (e.g. greater than or equal to three teeth with likely pulpal involvement).

- Insufficient coronal tooth tissue to ensure an effective coronal seal post-treatment.
- Caries involving the pulp chamber or root canal.

The Root Anatomy of Primary Molar Teeth

Paediatric dentists have traditionally favoured pulpotomy as opposed to complete extirpation of the pulp (pulpectomy) because of several perceived difficulties relating to the anatomy of the primary dentition. These are reported as:
- Ribbon shaped canals (difficult to instrument).
- Thin walls to canals (relative increase risk of perforation).
- Many lateral and furcal communications (difficult to clean and obturate).
- Physiological apical root resorption (wide open apical regions).
- Close proximity of the permanent tooth germ to the apex of primary tooth (relative risk of damaging successor tooth).

To Begin...

> *It is essential to provide adequate local anaesthesia before pulp treating a vital primary tooth.*

Additionally, it is worth remembering that even a tooth that appears to be completely non-vital may still have vital pulp tissue remaining. Therefore, it is essential that adequate pain relief is administered to ensure the continuing comfort and cooperation of the child. Effective moisture control is also important (ideally with dental dam where possible) for caries removal and any subsequent pulp therapy. If placement of dental dam is not achieved, dry guards, cotton wool rolls and a saliva ejector must be used once the pulp chamber is breached.

Pulp Therapy Techniques

The basic pulp therapy techniques available are dependant on the extent of pulpal inflammation and as such can be broadly divided into:
- **Pulp Capping** -This involves two approaches; direct and indirect. The direct pulp cap is not routinely used in the primary dentition.
- **Pulpotomy** - This can be performed on vital teeth, but the technique can differ in respect of choice of medicament and the number of visits required.

- **Pulpectomy** - This can be used for non-vital teeth with or without signs of infection. Complete extirpation of the pulp of a primary tooth and obturation with a resorbable material is gaining in popularity.

The common pulp therapy techniques available, the agents that can be used and the likely number of visits required are given (Figs 7-6 and 7-7). The management of a bleeding carious exposure (vital) is shown in Fig 7-6. The options for managing a carious exposure that does not bleed (non-vital) is shown in Fig 7-7.

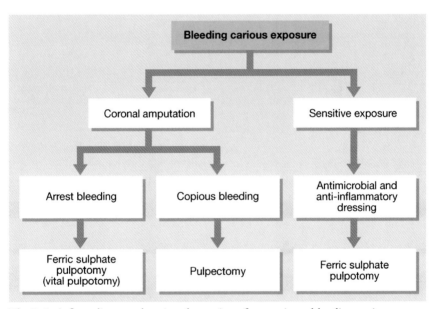

Fig 7-6 A flow diagram showing the options for treating a bleeding carious exposure in a primary tooth

Pulp Capping
Also termed indirect pulp therapy, this is used in the primary dentition to maintain vital pulp tissue. Pulp capping in the primary dentition may be divided into two different techniques:
- indirect
- direct.

Indirect pulp capping in primary molars
Also termed indirect pulp therapy, this involves placing a lining onto deep,

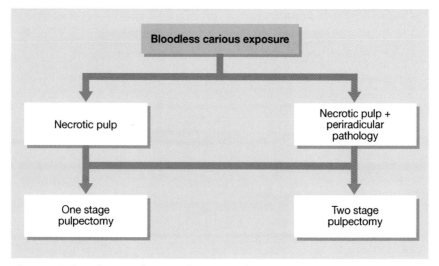

Fig 7-7 A flow diagram showing the options for treating a bloodless carious exposure in a primary tooth.

softened dentine in order to eliminate microbes and stimulate reparative secondary dentine and maintain pulp vitality. The technique is thought to be successful in pulp treatment of reversible inflammation in primary teeth with deep dentine caries.

Indirect pulp therapy technique
- The primary tooth must be symptom-free.
- The walls of cavity must be rendered caries-free, to permit sealing of the cavity margin.
- Deep, softened dentine may be left at the floor of the cavity, if its removal risks pulp exposure in a symptom-free tooth.
- There must be no evidence of pulpal exposure:
  - remove all caries from cavity walls
  - excavate cavity floor carefully
  - leave softened dentine, or thin layer of hard dentine, but do not expose the pulp
  - place a setting calcium hydroxide or a glass-ionomer cement lining over the stained or thin dentine
  - place a permanent, well-sealed restoration (compomer, preformed metal crown)
  - provide regular clinical and radiographic review.

Direct pulp capping in primary molars
This involves placing an agent directly onto a small traumatic pulpal exposure in order to stimulate the formation of a calcific barrier at the exposure site. This acts to protect the pulp tissue adjacent to the barrier. This approach should never be used for a carious exposure.
A direct pulp cap should only be used for pinpoint exposures caused by instrumentation. In paediatric dentistry, this may sometimes arise (although rarely) if a child unwittingly bites down on a bur during cavity preparation.

If a primary tooth has a carious exposure, the preferred method of treatment is a pulpotomy because infected and irreversibly inflamed coronal pulp should be removed. If there is a small area of contact between a calcium hydroxide direct pulp cap and an inflamed pulp, it will be ineffective, resulting in persistent inflammation, pulp death and often internal resorption. When calcium hydroxide is used as a direct pulp cap over a small exposure of healthy pulp tissue it can stimulate the deposition of a dentine barrier.

Direct pulp capping technique
- Arrest bleeding with gentle pressure from a sterile pledget of cotton wool moistened with saline (0.9%) placed over the exposure for 1-2 minutes.
- Bleeding must stop.
- Gently place a thin sub-lining of setting calcium hydroxide over the exposure and extend this to cover the adjacent dentine.
- Place a lining such as zinc oxide-eugenol or glass-ionomer cement over the sub-lining
- Permanently restore.
- Provide regular clinical and radiographic review.

Primary Molar Pulpotomy
In the primary dentition, pulp amputation or pulpotomy involves the removal of the coronal portion of the pulp, leaving residual pulp tissue *in-situ* in the root canals. The relative success of pulpotomy procedures in the primary dentition is illustrated in Fig 7-8.

The Ferric Sulphate Vital Pulpotomy

Classically, this involves the removal of irreversibly inflamed and infected coronal pulp tissue, leaving the uninflamed radicular pulp tissue *in-situ*. Clinically, the coronal pulp will bleed vigorously because it is hyperaemic — this is amputated, leaving vital, gently bleeding radicular pulp stumps, which should stop bleeding after two to three minutes. If bleeding stops, the tissue

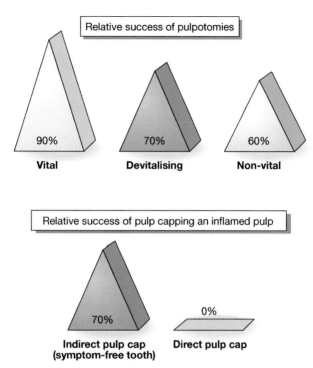

Fig 7-8 The relative success of pulpotomies in primary molar teeth. The devitalising and non-vital pulpotomies are no longer advocated since the removal of Buckley's Formocresol from use.

is assumed to possess the ability to recover from both the insult of caries and the amputation. If the bleeding does not stop there is irreversible inflammation and pulpectomy should be performed (Fig 7-9).

The now outmoded application of formocresol solution (even in its 20% dilute formulation) did not allow the radicular pulp tissue to heal, but instead widespread fixation occured along a gradient, which was greatest near the point of application. Some studies have shown that vital pulp tissue may remain apically. Despite this, the technique that used formocresol should be classed as one that rendered the radicular pulp non-vital. Ferric sulphate (15.5% formulation), an alternative to formocresol that is gaining in popularity, has shown good clinical success rates. When applied to a bleeding tissue the ferric and sulphate ions agglutinate with blood proteins to form a mechanical barrier at the ends of cut blood vessels, causing a styptic effect.

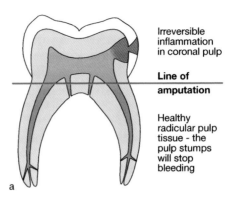

Irreversible
inflammation
in coronal pulp

Line of
amputation

Healthy
radicular pulp
tissue - the
pulp stumps
will stop
bleeding

Fig 7-9a The ideal scenario for vital pulpotomy.

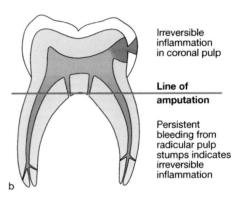

Irreversible
inflammation
in coronal pulp

Line of
amputation

Persistent
bleeding from
radicular pulp
stumps indicates
irreversible
inflammation

Fig 7-9b Vital pulpotomy would have a poor prognosis here.

It does not possess fixative properties and its antimicrobial properties, if any, are unknown.

Single-visit vital ferric sulphate pulpotomy technique (Fig 7-10)

- In pulpotomy procedures it is important to remove all caries and assess the degree of coronal destruction before embarking on pulp amputation. Once access to the pulp has been achieved, it is also important to use instruments and irrigant solutions that are sterile (Fig 7-11a).
- Prepare access cavity, extending to ensure complete removal of the roof of the pulp chamber. A non-end cutting bur (e.g. Batt bur) avoids perforating the thin floor of the pulp chamber (Fig 7-11b).
- Amputate the coronal pulp with excavators or slowly rotating round steel bur. Avoid perforating the thin pulp floor and remove all the coronal pulp tissue (Fig 7-11c).

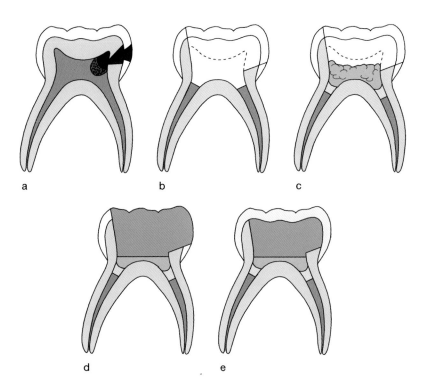

Fig 7-10 The single-visit ferric sulphate pulpotomy. (a) Cariously exposed primary molar. Irreversible inflammation and necrosis of pulp tissue exposed to caries. Caries removal will expose coronal pulp tissue. (b) Removal of caries and good access to the pulp chamber. Coronal pulp amputated leaving arrested bleeding sites indicative of uninflamed radicular pulp. (c) A 15% ferric sulphate solution applied to pulp stumps for 15 seconds via a cotton wool pledget or via a proprietary applicator. (d) Cotton wool removed, tooth restored with zinc oxide–eugenol cement directly over pulp stumps, then glass-ionomer cement. (e) A preformed metal crown is the definitive restoration. Note the haemostatic reaction within the coronal aspect of the radicular pulp tissue.

- Irrigate with saline (0.9%) or sterile water.
- Apply light pressure to pulp stumps with small pledget of cotton wool moistened with saline for three to four minutes (Fig 7-11d).
- If bleeding stops within three to four minutes, proceed. If not, consider removing further pulp tissue with an excavator or pulpectomy. Persistent bleeding is a sign of irreversible inflammation.

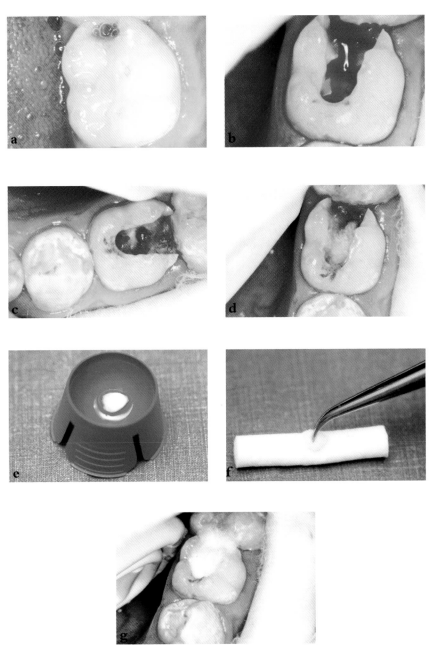

Fig 7-11 The clinical stages of the ferric sulphate pulpotomy for a primary molar.

- Place a small pledget of cotton wool into a drop of 15% ferric sulphate solution and blot this on fresh cotton wool or gauze. The cotton wool pledget should not be soaked (to avoid seepage onto the gingiva) but moistened with ferric sulphate (Fig 7-11e, f).
- Place the cotton wool pledget, moist with ferric sulphate, in gentle contact with the pulp stumps for 15 seconds (Fig 7-11g).
- In primary incisors, place a large paper point (moistened in a similar manner) in contact with the pulp stump.
- Remove the dressing after 15 seconds and assess whether pulpal bleeding has stopped. If bleeding continues, consider a second application of ferric sulphate.
- Restore with a setting zinc oxide-eugenol lining and restore with a permanent restoration affording good coronal seal (e.g. preformed metal crown).
- In primary incisors, a resorbable intracanal filler is required (e.g. pure zinc oxide powder mixed with eugenol liquid). This can be placed with a spiral filler if a thin paste, or packed down the canal with a paper point if a thicker paste is used.
- Provide regular clinical and radiographic review.

The Calcium Hydroxide Pulpotomy

Calcium hydroxide powder has also been used as an alternative to formocresol in vital pulpotomy. In the past, clinicians have used many different calcium hydroxide preparations, with varying results. Pure calcium hydroxide powder appears to be a useful agent, provided bleeding from the radicular pulp stumps stops. The powder is packed directly over the pulp stumps and the tooth is permanently restored.

Indications
These are similar to those cited for ferric sulphate pulpotomy. However, the following points should be adhered to strictly:
- The tooth must be symptom-free.
- The pulp should be vital.
- Coronal amputation must be achieved before the powder is placed in contact with the pulp tissue.
- Bleeding from the amputated radicular pulp stumps must not be copious and prolonged.

Technique
The stages of the technique are identical to the vital ferric sulphate pulpotomy up to achieving amputation. After which:

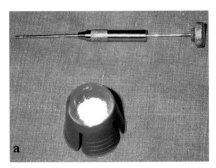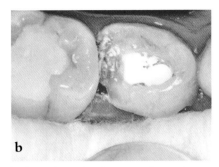

Fig 7-12 The clinical stages of the calcium hydroxide vital pulpotomy for a primary molar.

- Place a layer of well-condensed calcium hydroxide powder directly over the pulp stumps. The powder can be delivered to the tooth using a retrograde amalgam carrier (Fig 7-12a).
- Pack the powder well using small pledgets of dry, sterile cotton wool (Fig 7-12b).
- Place a lining of fast setting zinc oxide-eugenol cement directly over the calcium hydroxide layer.
- Restore as discussed previously.

Success
There has been little published on the efficacy of pure calcium hydroxide powder, but a study which compared this preparation with a dilute solution of formocresol in vital pulpotomy showed comparable success rates with both medicaments. It is worth noting, however, that the study only included cariously exposed vital primary molars which were symptom-free at presentation. The good success rates seen for calcium hydroxide in this study were probably because only teeth with healthy radicular pulps were included.

Dentine Bridge Formation
Calcium hydroxide is known to favour dentine deposition if placed over a pulp that is not irreversibly inflamed. Dentine bridge formation in response to the calcium hydroxide can be seen following its use as a pulpotomy agent in cariously exposed primary teeth. This indicates that the pulp has been successful at "walling itself off" from the irritant effects of the calcium hydroxide. The pulp tissue beneath the dentine barrier can maintain vital-

105

ity. Therefore the calcium hydroxide pulpotomy seeks to allow healing within a radicular pulp, rather than the fix the pulp as is seen following formocresol.

Caution

The presence of a dentine bridge beneath a calcium hydroxide pulpotomy in a primary molar does not indicate healing *per se*. The pulpotomy may fail, even in the presence of a dentine barrier. Electron microscopy studies have shown dentine barriers to be porous and therefore not true barriers to the ingress of microbes. Calcium hydroxide is highly alkaline, and this will irritate the cells of the pulp. The pulp must be able to react to this insult and remain vital beneath the layer of reactionary or "irritation" dentine.

* *In vital pulps, successful management and treatment outcome is dependent upon correct diagnosis.*
* *Pulpotomy itself will not result in pathological resorption, but inappropriate technique, poor coronal seal or deficient amputation can potentiate this.*

Desensitising Pulpotomy

Historically, this two-stage technique used paraformaldehyde paste to fix and devitalise the coronal and radicular pulp tissue. Pastes such as Aeslick's or Miller's are no longer used, therefore an alternative is suggested below.

Indications

* A tooth with a carious exposure of vital pulp, but a ferric sulphate pulpotomy cannot be carried out because the child will not accept local anaesthesia.
* Alternatively, local anaesthesia has been administered, but is inadequate for pulp amputation (hyperalgaesic pulp).

A steroidal antibiotic paste (e.g. Ledermix™) is placed gently over the exposure site. This may kill microbes and reduce inflammation. The larger the exposure, the more profound the effect of reducing pulp sensitivity.

Two-stage desensitising pulpotomy technique

First visit
* Irrigate exposure site with sterile saline (0.9%) and gently dry with cotton wool pledgets (Fig 7-13a).

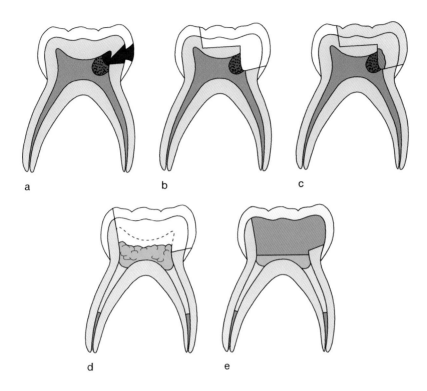

Fig 7-13 The desensitising pulpotomy.

- Pulp exposure following caries removal. The pulp is vital and very sensitive — vital pulpotomy cannot be attempted (Fig 7-13b).
- Place a small pledget of cotton wool loaded with paste directly over the exposure site. Do not apply excess pressure, as this is thought to precipitate pain.
- Anchor the cotton wool with a setting calcium hydroxide lining material.
- Place a well-sealed temporary restoration and leave for seven to 14 days (Fig 7-13c).

Second visit
- If the initial exposure site was large, the pulp tissue (at least coronally)

should be less sensitive. Administer local anaesthesia and proceed to a ferric sulphate pulpotomy (Fig 7-13d).

- If the coronal pulp remains sensitive, enlargement of the exposure site may be carried out with further application of paste.
- A preformed metal crown is the definitive restoration (Fig 7-13e).

Success rate

The devitalising pulpotomy using paraformaldehyde was not as successful as the single-visit pulpotomy: it had an approximate success rate of 70%. There is little published data on the use of Ledermix™ in the primary dentition.

Pulpectomy

Pulpectomy techniques in the primary dentition are gaining in popularity and will become more widespread now that formocresol is no longer available for use in non-vital pulpotomy techniques.

Success rate

Non-vital pulpotomy was not as successful as either the vital or devitalising techniques, with an approximate success rate of 60%. The success rate of pulpectomy has yet to be investigated fully, with very few large scale studies. Despite this, it is becoming the preferred treatment over pulpotomy in some countries.

Indications
- Irreversible inflammation evident in radicular pulp tissue, shown by persistent bleeding at the radicular pulp stumps after coronal amputation.
- Completely non-vital radicular pulp with or without signs of infection.

Pulpectomy technique
There are two methods of approaching a pulpectomy, depending on whether the radicular pulp is irreversibly inflamed (copious bleeding even after removal of the ferric sulphate) or non-vital (no bleeding) (Fig 7-14). This can be assessed only after coronal pulp amputation.

One-visit pulpectomy: irreversible radicular pulpitis (canal debridement only)
This is indicated for a radicular pulp that will not stop bleeding and is irreversibly inflamed. The process involves cleaning the root canals without attempting to shape.
- Identify root canals
- Irrigate with an effective irrigant solution, such as sodium hypochlorite solu-

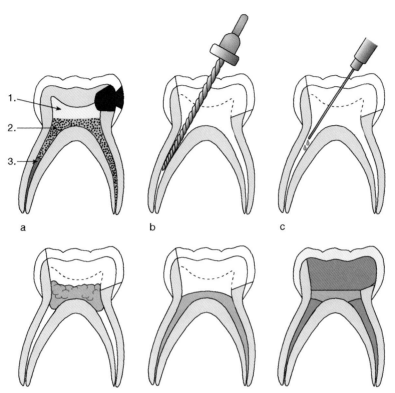

Fig 7-14 The pulpectomy. (a) A cariously exposed primary molar with areas of necrotic pulp (1), irreversible inflammation (2) and some residual vital tissue (3). (b) Identify root canals using a radiograph. Insert small files into root canals, keeping 2mm from the radiographic apex. Lightly and gently clean walls of canal but do not shape. (c) Copious irrigation with hypochlorite solution. Dry canals with premeasured paper points. (d) If the root canals are wet with exudate, consider injecting non-setting calcium hydroxide paste into the canals. Place a dry pledget of cotton wool in pulp chamber and restore temporarily for seven to 14 days. This can be left *in-situ* for seven to 14 days before obturating. (e) If the canals are dry, or if there is evidence of healing after seven to 14 days, obturate root canals with a slow-setting paste (e.g. pure zinc oxide-eugenol) using a spiral paste filler or blunt end of a paper point. (f) Restore as for vital pulpotomy.

tion (0.5-1%) or chlorhexidine solution (0.4%) to clear debris. Insert small files (no greater than size 30) into canals, keeping 2mm short of the radiographic apex. File canal walls lightly and gently, irrigate again to remove debris. Do not remove dentine (i.e. "shape"), as the canal walls are very thin.

• Dry canals with a premeasured paper point, (remaining 2mm from the apices)

- Obturate with slow-setting paste (e.g. slow-setting pure zinc oxide-eugenol) using spiral paste filler or packing with the blunt end of a paper point.
- Place a well-sealed permanent restoration as before.

Two-visit pulpectomy: non-vital teeth
This technique is best reserved for those teeth that are non-vital but may also have an associated chronic sinus (infection). The initial cleaning and dressing serves to treat any infection that may be present.

Visit one (extirpation, cleaning and dressing)
- The steps are identical to the one-visit pulpectomy.
- Dress the tooth with non-setting calcium hydroxide paste and seal with a dry cotton wool pledget and setting zinc oxide-eugenol cement. Consider prescribing a systemic antimicrobial.

Visit two (obturation and coronal restoration)
If healing has occured the steps involved are identical to the latter stages of the one-visit pulpectomy. If healing has not occured, extraction is indicated.

Once pulp therapy has been undertaken it is essential that the child is reviewed on a regular basis, both clinically and radiographically. After undergoing pulp treatment, carers should be advised to return if any symptoms arise from their child's tooth.

Clinical and Radiographic Review

Clinical Review
The tooth should be monitored clinically perhaps one month postoperatively, then subsequently at six-monthly intervals. Successful clinical outcome can be marked by:
- A pain free pulp-treated tooth.
- Absence of any signs or symptoms of periapical infection, such as
  - tenderness to percussion
  - buccal/lingual/palatal tenderness or swelling
  - sinus formation and associated mobility.

Radiographic Review
Generally, it is recommended that any tooth that has undergone endodon-

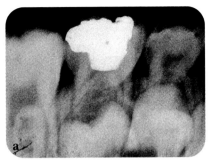 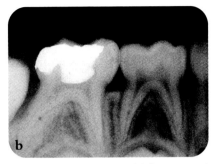

Fig 7-15 Radiographic views of successful vital pulpotomies using (a) formocresol and (b) calcium hydroxide powder approximately one year after treatment.

tic treatment is assessed using annual radiographs (bitewings will suffice. Fig 7-15). Successful radiographic outcome can by marked by:

• Normal exfoliation of the pulpotomised tooth.
• Absence of periradicular pathology.
• Absence of internal resorption.
• Normal eruption of the permanent successor.

The Formocresol Controversy has Ended

The medicament that was advocated up until June 2004 for application onto the radicular pulp stumps for a vital or non-vital pulpotomy was a 1:5 dilution of Buckley's formocresol. This solution was also used during pulpectomy procedures.

Formocresol contains formaldehyde, which is a potent antimicrobial agent and tissue fixative. It also contains tricresol, which is antimicrobial, though role in formocresol is unclear.

The technique of vital pulp therapy has been used in primary teeth since the 1950s with much success. The dilute solution was advocated for use in the 1970s and is as effective as the full-strength solution. Success rates ranging from 80–100% were reported.

There was growing concern, however, over the safety of even a 1:5 dilution of formocresol, centred on one of its constituents, formaldehyde which is soluble in water, highly reactive and metabolised rapidly. The following effects have been cited in human case reports and laboratory-based animal or cell culture studies.

Local Effects
- Soft-tissue burns.
- Disordered formation of underlying tooth germ (reported in human case studies).
- Disturbance of eruption of the permanent successor tooth (reported in human case studies).

General Effects
Formocresol has a rapid systemic distribution (reported in primates and canine studies) and is known to have mutagenic and carcinogenic potential (reported in primates, cell culture and rats studies) as well as being embryotoxic and teratogenic (reported in studies using chick embryos).

Radioisotope-labelled formaldehyde has been identified systemically in the following tissues in dogs after multiple formocresol pulpotomies:
- Periodontal ligament, bone, dentine and pulp.
- Liver, lungs and kidney.
- Brain.

However, within paediatric dentistry, the decision to abandon the use of formocresol was finally made following a release from the IARC in June 2004. This document stated that formaldehyde vapour is a carcinogen in humans. The large, systematic review concluded from serveral extended cohort studies that formaldehyde has a positive correlation with nasopharyngeal carcinoma and possibly other upper respiratory tract sites such as the nasal mucosa and paranasal sinuses. The alternative agent that some teaching centres have begun using is ferric sulphate.

Alternatives to Formocresol
Several agents/techniques have been evaluated as possible alternatives to the formocresol vital pulpotomy. These include:
- Calcium hydroxide pastes, cements and powder.
- Electrosurgery.
- Lasers.
- Ferric sulphate.
- Bone-morphogenic proteins.
- Mineral trioxide aggregate.

Although some of these agents/techniques prove promising, there has been insufficient clinical research involving these alternatives. Formocresol was the "gold standard" of pulpotomy agents but can no longer be advocated. One of the reasons why it was so successful, even in inexperienced hands, was because it could "deal" with an inflamed radicular pulp better than any of its alternatives. It will fix an inflamed pulp, whereas alternatives such as calcium hydroxide and ferric sulphate and mineral trioxide aggregate are unable to produce fixation, but rely more upon allowing the pulp to heal. The bottom line is that, even in this modern age, we are still unable to promote healing in an irreversible pulpitis. Despite this, there have been promising early results from calcium hydroxide powder, ferric sulphate solution, and mineral trioxide aggregate. With these alternative medicaments it is generally thought that they have a greater chance of success if there is no inflammation (or mild reversible inflammation) present within the radicular pulp. Clinical trials looking at these agents (particularly ferric sulphate) are increasing but further research is required to assess long-term survival rates, effects upon pulp tissue and the possibility of systemic distribution.

Internal Resorption – Is There An Increased Risk Following Pulp Therapy?

Present-day thinking suggests that the inflammatory status of the residual pulp tissue has greatest bearing upon a successful outcome following vital pulpotomy. If the radicular pulp stumps are bleeding copiously and prolonged, vital pulp therapy techniques should not be used. The tooth should be treated with a pulpectomy.

In vital pulpotomy, it follows logically, that if ferric sulphate or calcium hydroxide is used on an irreversibly inflamed radicular pulp, healing will not occur. Chronic inflammation will ensue, leading to a greater risk of internal resorption. Chronic inflammation will stimulate odontoclastic activity within the pulp system, producing pathological resorption.

Instruments And Medicaments

Table 7-1 outlines the basic instruments and restorative materials required for a range of pulp therapy treatment for primary teeth. It is worthwhile noting that the armamentarium is simple and most of the items are very readily obtainable.

Table 7-1 **The basic instruments and restorative materials for pulp therapy**

Procedure	Instrument/medicament
Cavity outline and caries removal	• Small high-speed diamond burs (fissure and round) • Small slow-speed steel burs (no. 1 and 2 round)
Unroofing the pulp chamber	• Dental dam • Non-end-cutting fissure bur (e.g. Batt bur)
Coronal pulp amputation	• Sterile sharp excavators • Sterile round steel bur (e.g. no. 2)
Stop bleeding at radicular pulp stumps	• Small sterile pledgets of cotton wool • Sterile saline or water in an endodontic syringe
Root canal instrumentation (pulpectomy)	• Small endodontic files with rubber stops to control the working length • Irrigant solution (e. g. hypochlorite or chlorhexidine solution) in an endodontic syringe • Paper points (measured to working length)
Root canal obturation (pulpectomy)	• Slow-setting pure zinc oxide-eugenol cement • Spiral paste fillers, or pack paste with the blunt end of a paper point
Restoration of pulp chamber	• Fast setting zinc oxide-eugenol cement
Intracoronal restoration	• Glass-ionomer cement or compomer with appropriate bonding agent
Extra coronal restoration	• Preformed metal crown with glass ionomer luting cement

Medicaments

The commonly used pulp therapy medicaments are described below.

Ferric sulphate 15% solution

Astringedent™ Ferric sulphate 15% in aqueous vehicle.

Stronger solutions are available but are not indicated for pulp therapy. It can be applied using cotton wool, or a special applicator.

Ledermix™ paste

1 gram of paste contains:

active ingredients
    Triamcinolone acetonide (steroid)   10mg
    Demeclocycline (antimicrobial)   30mg

also contains
    calcium chloride
    zinc oxide
    sodium sulphite
    triethanolamine
    polyethyleneglycols
    purified water

Practical Tips

- The reasons for failure often fall into one or more of these categories:
  - poor choice of teeth
  - inadequate pulp amputation
  - coronal leakage.

- Radiographs should be taken before a decision is made to perform pulp therapy.
- Local anaesthesia should be administered wherever possible. In the mandible, infiltrations can be used until eruption of the first permanent molar.
- A common exposure site is the high mesial pulp horn.
- Use a small sharp excavator to remove the last fragments of coronal pulp tissue. Avoid the use of burs on the floor of the pulp chamber; it is thin and liable to perforate.
- Blot the ferric sulphate-moist cotton wool pledget before placing it over the amputation site. Place dry cotton wool over the top of this to prevent seepage onto soft tissues, even if you have dental dam placed.
- Place a good, long-lasting restoration post pulp treatment, ideally a preformed metal crown.

References

Barr ES, Flaitz CM, Hicks MJ. A retrospective radiographic evaluation of primary molar pulpectomies. Pediatric Dentistry 1991;13:4-9.

Casas MJ, Kenny DJ, Johnston DH, Judd PL. Long-term outcomes of primary molar ferric sulfate pulpotomy and root canal therapy. Pediatric Dentistry 2004;26:44-48.

Eidelman E, Holan G, Fuks AB. Mineral trioxide aggregate vs. formocresol in pulpotomized primary molars: A preliminary report. Pediatric Dentistry 2001;23:15-18.

Farooq NS, Coll JA, Kuwabara A, Shelton P. Success rates of formocresol pulpotomy and indirect pulp therapy in the treatment of deep dentinal caries in primary teeth. Pediatric Dentistry 2000;22:278-286.

Fuks AB. Current concepts in vital primary pulp therapy. European Journal of Paediatric Dentistry 2002;3:115-120.

Hobson P. Pulp treatment of deciduous teeth. Part 2: Clinical investigation. Br Dental J 1970;128:275-283.

International Agency for Research on Cancer. IARC classifies formaldehyde as carcinogenic to humans. Press Release No 153. http://www.iarc.fr/pageroot/PRELEASES/pr153a.html.

Smith NL, Seale NS, Nunn ME. Ferric sulfate pulpotomy in primary molars: A retrospective study. Pediatric Dentistry 2000;22:192-199.

Waterhouse PJ. Formocresol and alternative primary molar pulpotomy medicaments. A review. Endodon Dent Traumatol 1995;11:157-162.

Waterhouse PJ, Nunn JH, Whitworth JM. An investigation of the relative efficacy of Buckley's formocresol and calcium hydroxide in primary molar vital pulp therapy. Br Dental J 2000;188:32–36.

Chapter 8
Avoiding Extraction of Carious Anterior Primary Teeth

Aim

The aim of this chapter is to discuss the techniques available to restore anterior primary teeth.

Outcome

After reading this chapter the practitioner should have knowledge of the different approaches to restoring caries in anterior teeth. In addition, you should have awareness that many of the techniques covered in this chapter are simple to provide, using equipment and materials that are easily obtainable.

Introduction

Dental caries affecting the anterior primary teeth can have a major impact upon a child's appearance (Fig 8-1) and, to this end, parents may seek the help of a dentist in order to improve their child's appearance. Treatment depends upon the extent of the carious destruction and the age and level of cooperation of the child. It is worth noting that, ideally, most paediatric dentists would treat caries in the posterior teeth before the anterior, since the primary molars are important in maintaining arch length. Despite this, there

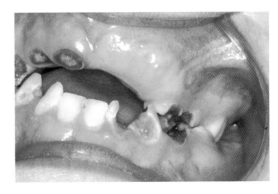

Fig 8-1 The primary dentition of a young child with rampant caries.

119

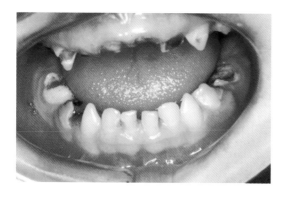

Fig 8-2 Early childhood caries caused by sugary liquids in a feeding bottle – "nursing" or "bottle" caries.

is some value in treating small anterior lesions first in a treatment plan involving acclimatisation. Improving anterior aesthetics in a child may also boost the willingness of both the parents/carers and the child to cooperate with any planned preventive programme.

Carious Lesions In Primary Anterior Teeth

In very young children — those of preschool age — the presence of caries in the upper anterior teeth is often due to a condition known as early childhood caries, previously termed "nursing caries" (Fig 8-2). Prolonged and frequent drinking of liquids high in non-milk extrinsic sugars usually cause it. These drinks are often given to the child via a nursing bottle or feeder-cup, particularly at sleep-time, allowing sugary liquid to pool around the anterior teeth. In severe cases, the posterior teeth may also be involved. Early childhood caries or nursing caries in young children can be aggressive and develop rapidly, resulting in gross coronal destruction. The carious destruction in such cases often begins with a labial lesion (Class V), which may then become confluent with approximal (Class III) lesions — resulting in a large circumferential lesion.

School -aged children may also develop carious anterior teeth, but lesions tend to be less aggressive than nursing caries and of a different distribution, with approximal lesions (Class III) common.

It is less common to see dental caries affecting the lower anterior primary teeth. These teeth benefit from being constantly bathed in saliva from the submandibular and sublingual glands, and the tongue acts to cover these teeth when infants drink from a bottle or feeder cup. If caries is present at this site, a diagnosis of rampant caries is appropriate.

The Proximal Lesion
- This lesion starts at the site of the broad contact area.
- A common site appears to be the mesial surface of the primary incisors.
- In the mixed dentition the distal aspect of primary canines can be affected, particularly if there is contact between the canine and first primary molar (no primate space).
- If left untreated, the proximal lesion will undermine the incisal edge relatively quicker than would occur in the permanent dentition because of the shorter crown length of the primary tooth.

Caries involving enamel should be treated by a package of preventive measures (not just topical fluoride application). Once dentine is involved, restorative treatment should be provided. When a decision has been made to remove the caries, should the tooth be left "self-cleansing" by using the method of discing, or will cavity preparation be required with subsequent restoration?

Discing
This is a useful technique to treat proximal lesions, which have not involved the pulp. It requires full or partial caries removal proximally, leaving either a crown with parallel sides mesially and distally or gently tapering towards the incisal edge. This approach is most appropriate in children older than three years, since the upper canines are fully erupted by this age. Once the primary canines are erupted it is thought that reduction in the mesiodistal width of the primary incisal edges will not result in space loss.

- *Discing removes superficial caries only, leaving any remaining caries in a self-cleansing area.*

- *It relies upon compliance with a preventive programme to be successful, since the aim is to promote arrest of residual caries.*

- *Although this technique is extremely useful, aesthetics can be poor.*

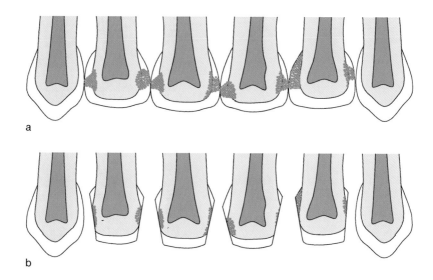

Fig 8-3 (a) Approximal caries (not involving the pulp) in maxillary primary incisors. (b) Maxillary primary incisors after discing. The teeth appear tapered and are not caries free. The disced areas should be self-cleansing. Topical fluoride may be applied to the disced areas at this stage.

The amount of tooth removal is limited by the close proximity of the pulp horns. A high fluoride concentration varnish (e.g. Duraphat™) can be applied after discing to promote remineralisation (Fig 8-3).

Useful instruments (Fig 8-4)
- Small abrasive discs ranging from coarse to fine.
- Mandrel.
- Slow handpiece.
- A tapered bur maybe an alterative instrument.

Access
The discs are placed interproximally in order to remove superficial caries. It is vitally important that the patient's lips and tongue are retracted to avoid iatrogenic injury. This can be achieved with cotton wool rolls (lips) and a small saliva ejector (tongue) and the dentist's fingers!

Caries removal
The aim of this technique is to make the tooth's incisal edge narrower in a

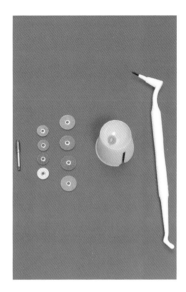

Fig 8-4 Miniature abrasive polishing discs and small mandrel used for safer discing. Topical fluoride varnish can be applied to the disced areas with a brush.

mesiodistal aspect than its cervical width - to produce a "self-cleansing" area. The site of the lesion dictates the angulation of the disc at the tooth surface. If caries is deep, do not attempt to remove it with the disc, since pulpal exposure will occur. Aim for parallel sides or a gentle taper mesiodistally. Smooth sharp line angles with the finer grades of abrasive disc.

Fluoride application
Some paediatric dentists favour application of a varnish containing a high fluoride concentration to the prepared approximal surfaces to aid arrest of caries.

Practical Tips: Discing

- This technique must be used in conjunction with preventive programme involving dietary advice and oral hygiene instruction.
- It is wise to discuss the resulting shape of the teeth before you embark on discing.
- Miniature abrasive discs are available and lessen the potential for soft-tissue damage.
- Avoid metal polishing strips or discs. They generate excessive amounts of heat and may cause gingival trauma.

Cavity Preparation (Class III)
When caries is well into dentine, but not involving the pulp, cavity preparation and restoration should be done instead of discing. This will give a better aesthetic result.

Useful instruments
- Small sharp excavators.
- Slow speed - sizes 1 and 2 round steel burs.
- High speed - pear shaped and small round diamond burs.

Access
This can depend on whether the anterior tooth proximal contacts are open or closed.
- Closed — access may be gained via the buccal (mandibular teeth) or palatal (maxillary teeth) aspect at the level of the mid-third of the crown. Small round steel or diamond burs are useful to gain access.
- Open — access achieved more easily directly via interproximal surface using small round steel burs, or small excavators.

Caries removal
- Avoiding unnecessary destruction of sound tooth tissue, the cavity outline will be dictated by caries removal but will probably be "C" shaped. Again, round steel burs are used to remove caries.
- Internal angles should be rounded to avoid pulp exposure.

Restoration
- A lining of hard-setting calcium hydroxide may be placed on the axial wall as an indirect pulp cap. However, glass-ionomer-type lining agents (e.g. Vitrebond) may be placed directly on the axial wall of the cavity.
- In anterior dentitions with closed contacts, cellulose matrix strips must be used to ensure contacts and embrasures remain patent.
- A glass-ionomer restoration may be used because of its adhesive and possible fluoride-releasing properties. However, aesthetically it is quite opaque.
- More translucent materials such as composite or compomer may also be used if the child can tolerate the use of bonding systems and more stringent moisture control.
- Special "paediatric" shades of composite are available to shade-match with the relatively lighter enamel of primary teeth.

The Buccal or Labial Lesion (Class V)
This lesion usually involves the gingival one-third of the labial surface of an

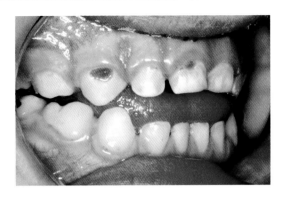

Fig 8-5 Buccal/labial caries affecting the maxillary primary canine and incisors.

incisor or canine and can be diagnosed by direct vision. They can be difficult to deal with if the carious lesion extends below the gingival margin (Fig 8-5).

Useful instruments
- Small sharp excavators.
- Slow speed - sizes 1 and 2 round steel burs.
- High speed - pear shaped and small round diamond burs.

Technique
In these lesions, caries appears to spread laterally to involve a large surface area of tooth tissue. Caries removal results in a cavity where there is much more dentine than enamel exposed. The enamel layer is relatively thin in cross-section at the cervical region of the tooth, so a cavity in this region will have more dentine than enamel available for bonding.

Access
Access is obviously direct for cavity preparation. Outline can be established using diamond burs.

Caries removal
The principles of preparation are similar to approximal lesions. Caries removal often produces a "sausage" or kidney-shaped cavity outline. Caries may be removed using a small round steel bur or a small sharp excavator.

Restoration
The choice of material for lining and restoring is similar to approximal lesions. However, the cavity affords little enamel and relatively more dentine available for bonding, so if glass-ionomer is not used, consider the use of a den-

125

tine-bonding agent prior to placing composite or compomer. Proprietary light-transmitting matrices (e.g. a Hawes Neos cervical matrix) can be used to contour the restoration and reduce polishing time.

Practical Tips

- Any areas of enamel decalcification or areas of enamel breakdown within 2 mm of the main lesion should be included in the main cavity preparation.
- Use a size 1 or 2 round steel bur to remove subgingival caries. Doing this you are reliant upon the "feel" of caries removal afforded by a slow hand-piece.
- There are now single-stage bonding systems available (e.g. Scotchbond 1), which simplify the stages of bonding.
- If a cervical matrix is not used, use a blunt, straight probe to ensure the restorative material is well packed and any excess restorative material is removed.

The Circumferential Lesion

A labial lesion may accompany an approximal lesion on the same tooth, so that the two lesions are in close proximity or merge. This can produce quite extensive coronal breakdown (Fig 8-6). Again, one needs to consider the required longevity of any proposed restoration and the age and level of co-operation of the child before a decision can be made as to whether to restore the tooth and, indeed, what restorative approach is best for the child. There are two restorative options available:

- A combination of discing and restoration.
- Placement of a composite "strip" crown.

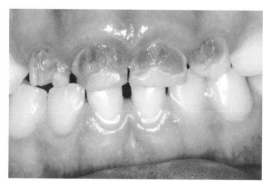

Fig 8-6 Circumferential carious lesions affecting the maxillary primary incisors.

Discing Plus Restoration

This technique involves discing the approximal lesion and removing caries from the labial lesion and restoring the labial surface only. Both these approaches have already been discussed, but the following points are noteworthy:

- This approach should be accompanied by a rigorous preventive package.
- Where the labial restoration meets the area of disced enamel there will be no margin for the restorative material. Here the restoration should be finished flush with the approximal preparation.
- The restoration will not possess resistance to lateral displacement, so bonding agents are recommended.

Composite Crowns

Caries removal will have rendered the tooth severely broken down. The following points may indicate the placement of a "direct" crown on a primary tooth:

- Gross coronal breakdown of a tooth still required to give several years more service.
- Post-pulpotomy/pulpectomy.
- Cooperative children with parents/carers who are extremely keen to maintain the primary dentition.

Technique

- Caries removal is dictated by the site of the lesion and may include labial and approximal circumferential lesions.
- Pulp therapy, if required, should be carried out before crown placement.
- If the pulp has not been exposed, but the axial wall of the cavity is close to the pulp, consider an indirect pulp cap with a hard-setting calcium hydroxide lining material before coronal restoration.

Materials required for coronal restoration:

- Multipurpose bonding agent (since you will be bonding to both enamel and dentine).
- An extra light or "paediatric" shade of hybrid composite resin.
- Celluloid crown formers for primary anterior teeth in a range of sizes.
- Abrasive polishing discs (e.g. small Soflex discs).
- Fine diamond composite finishing burs.
- Articulating paper.
- Scissors.

How to choose the correct crown former

Choosing the correct celluloid crown former is similar in principle to choos-

127

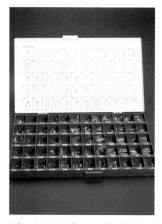

Fig 8-7 A box of celluloid crown formers.

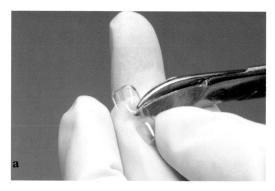

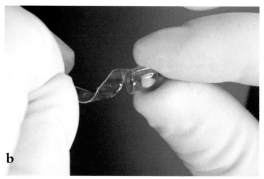

Fig 8-8 (a–b) A crown former being trimmed with Beebee scissors.

ing the correct preformed metal crown (stainless steel crown Fig 8-7). Basically, there are two methods:

- Measure the mesiodistal width of the incisal edge of the tooth using a pair of spring dividers and choose the nearest matching celluloid crown.
- Offer up the chosen celluloid crown, its incisal edge to the natural tooth's incisal edge and choose the best match (trial and error).

Customising the celluloid crown former

These always need trimming because the crown former usually also covers the root surface of each tooth (Fig 8-8):

- Measure the maximum length of the natural crown with a periodontal probe and trim the celluloid crown so that it is 1mm longer.
- Reproduce the natural contours of the gingival margin on the crown former (a "smile" labially and palatally, and a "frown" interproximally).
- Try the crown former on the tooth during trimming.

128

- Smooth any rough margins with scissors or slowly rotating sandpaper discs.
- Carefully place a vent hole at one of the incisal corners of the crown former using a straight probe. This allows air and a little excess composite resin to flow out of the former.

Coronal restoration
- Choose the appropriate shade of composite resin using a shade guide.
- Isolate the tooth to be restored.
- Apply the bonding system to all the coronal tissue (following the manufacturer's instructions).
- Place the composite resin into the crown form until it is 2/3 to 3/4 full. This depends on the amount of tooth tissue missing.
- Place the crown form firmly but slowly over the crown of the tooth, allowing any excess air and composite to escape through the venthole.
- Remove any gross excess of material from the margins and the vent hole.
- Polymerise with a dental curing light source for the recommended amount of time on each surface of the crown. This ensures an adequate depth of cure throughout.
- Using a small excavator or straight probe, carefully "strip" the crown form from the tooth.
- Check the occlusion with articulating paper and adjust as necessary using fine diamond finishing burs. Adjust the composite crown length if necessary.
- Check the margins of the composite crown with a straight probe and adjust any areas that are too bulky or overhanging, again using composite finishing burs or abrasive discs.

Practical Tips
- When trimming the crown form, cut a small amount at a time.
- If you attempt to cut a large slice off the celluloid, you run the risk of fracturing the former. It is quite brittle.
- Trim towards the incisal edge rather like peeling an orange – so that you end up with a "spiral" of trimmed crown former.
- When placing the vent hole using a straight probe, ensure your fingers are well away from where the probe will penetrate through the former.
- After restoring the crown, if you cannot remove the crown form it may be left *in-situ* providing the margins are very smooth and the length of the crown appropriate. The patient should be reviewed a week later and further attempt at removing the form should be made.

References

Fayle SA, Welbury RR, Roberts JF. British Society of Paediatric Dentistry: A policy document on management of caries in the primary dentition. Int J Paediatric Dent 2001;11:153-157.

Chapter 9
How to Cheat at Dental Dam

Aim

To demonstrate a simple, straight forward method of applying dental dam in the restorative management of children.

Outcome

On completing this chapter the practitioner should feel confident to use the split dam technique during operative dental treatment.

Introduction

All dental restoratives are moisture-sensitive, yet using dental dam is not something that the busy dental operator often considers when managing children. However, mastering a simple "cheat" such as the split dam technique achieves better access in small mouths and avoids cotton wool rolls.

Children often hate cotton wool rolls. They don't like water pooled under their tongue or in the retromolar area. They object to "bits" on their tongue and don't like the taste of many of the dental medicaments. Using dental dam solves these problems. The child who has a dental dam in the mouth is encouraged to keep their mouth open without the use of a mouth prop.

Dental dam is particularly useful for children with retching problems, especially when it is combined with nitrous oxide inhalation sedation. It keeps their tongue away from the operating area, reassures them that they will not choke on the materials and helps them feel more disassociated from the operative procedure. As such, it has a prominent role in the management of these children and should be attempted as an alternative to referral for general anaesthesia.

Advantages of Dental Dam

Dental dam isolation has many positive benefits:
• Reduced risk of cross-infection.

- Safer airway.
- Tongue, cheeks and lips are kept away from the operating area.
- No more struggling with wet cotton rolls.
- Operator has both hands free.
- Reduced child anxiety over choking or inhaling materials.
- More effective nitrous oxide inhalation sedation (since it encourages nose breathing).
- Reduced environmental contamination with nitrous oxide during sedation.

Dental Dam Myths

There are various reasons why dental dam (Fig 9-1) is not widely accepted in paediatric dental practice in the UK. Examples are as follows:
- Difficult to apply.
- Needs lots of equipment.
- Adds time to treatment.
- Not well tolerated.
- The child doesn't like it.
- Fear of latex allergy.

However, with practice, especially using a simple "split dam" technique, dental dam is not difficult to apply and, indeed, saves time in the long run. The simple technique outlined in this chapter requires only basic equipment and very few clamps. Furthermore, if the "tooth raincoat" is introduced suitably into the treatment plan, dentists will find that children prefer it to cotton rolls and like having a barrier between them and the operative procedure, medicaments and equipment. Silicone vinyl dam can be used to reduce risk of latex allergy.

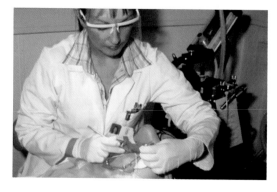

Fig 9-1 Dental dam is particularly useful when inhalation sedation is being used to encourage nose breathing and reduce environmental nitrous oxide.

The Bare Essentials

The basic equipment in a dental dam kit are (Fig 9-2):
- Dental dam (Fig 9-3) - thick or extra thick.
- Dental dam clamps:
    - Ash K (permanent molar).
    - Ash A (primary molar or permanent premolar).
    - Ash D (primary molar or permanent premolar).
- A single hole punch.
- A frame (metal is less bulky than plastic).
- A pair of scissors.

Isolating Anterior Teeth

- For best results, restoration of carious or traumatised incisors usually requires adequate moisture control.
- In the mixed dentition the anterior teeth have relatively poor contact points. Using a split dam to isolate all four anterior teeth helped by using elastic wedges is a simple means of isolating these teeth.
- Once the canines have erupted these can be incorporated into the split dam.

The Split Dam Technique: Anterior Teeth

- Punch two holes in the dental dam approximately 2-2.5cm apart (Fig 9-4).
- Make a slit by joining the two holes together (Fig 9-5).
- Put the chair as flat as it can go.
- Invite the child to raise the chin up "into the air".

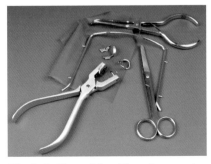

Fig 9-2 Essential rubber dam equipment.

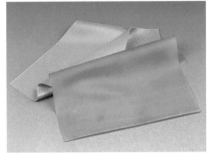

Fig 9-3 Dental dam is also available as "latex-free" (vinyl).

133

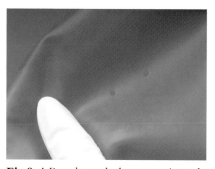

Fig 9-4 Punch two holes approximately 2cm apart.

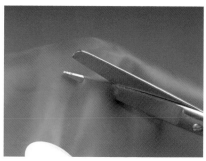

Fig 9-5 Make a slit by joining the holes together.

- Place cotton wool rolls under the upper lip.
- Dry the teeth.
- Place one end of the slit into the interproximal area at one end of the area to be isolated (either distal to the lateral incisor or distal to the canine).
- **Tip** - lead with the "sharp" edge of the dental dam into the interproximal area.
- Place wedjets if required (no clamps are needed).
- Keep either your mirror or your assistant's suction pressed against the dam (but not the roof of the mouth) in the anterior palate area.
- Invite the child to raise their hand if they need the saliva ejector ("if you're drowning, raise your hand and I'll place the sucky straw"), otherwise leave it out of the mouth since children tend to fiddle with it.

The Split Dam Technique: Posterior Teeth

This cheat technique does not give the complete isolation that the original methods bestow. Therefore, the occasional use of a saliva ejector, especially during air rota preparation, is to be recommended. However, the key benefit is in soft-tissue control, which greatly facilitates access and is a must for adhesive restorations and pulp therapy.

- Punch two holes in the dental dam approximately 2-2.5cm apart.
- Make a slit by joining the two holes together.
- Place a clamp (raincoat "clip" or "toggle") on the most posterior molar tooth, either first permanent molar or the second primary molar.
- Grab the dental dam firmly between first fingers and thumbs.
- Place over the bow of the clamp, then push downwards over the wings.
- Stretch the slit anteriorly and place between the anterior teeth (Fig 9-6).

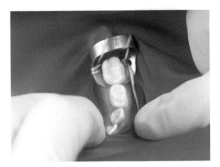

Fig 9-6 Place over the bow and downwards over the wings then stretch forwards and insert the edge between the most convenient anterior teeth.

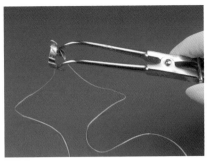

Fig 9-7 Take care to insert floss through both holes in the clamp to avoid aspiration.

- **Tip** - use the "sharp" edge of the dental dam to lead into the anterior interproximal space.
- Place the frame.

Handy Hints And Shortcuts

- Dry the teeth, otherwise the dental dam slips.
- Put floss through both holes and around the bow of the dental dam clamp to prevent aspiration, should it disengage (Fig 9-7).
- There are various proprietory accessories that are ready available through regular dental suppliers:
  - "Wedjets", useful to anchor the dam interproximally.
  - Preformed dam with an inbuilt frame, such as "Dry Dam".

Introducing Dental Dam To The Child

Children are always fearful of the unknown — whether it be a new dental environment, operator, technique or instrument — even if they are not otherwise considered to be dentally anxious. Therefore, appropriate introduction of dental dam to the child greatly improves its acceptability.
- Use child-friendly language to describe the dam and equipment.
- Reassure the child that the dental dam punch doesn't go into their mouth!
- Let the child see themselves (wearing the "Halloween mask") in a mirror following placement.
- Consider doing a restoration first without dental dam, then explain how using dam next time will prevent the use of cotton rolls (posteriorly) and "stops bits falling on the tongue".

Practical Tips

- Dry the teeth.
- Choose thick dental dam sheets.
- Introduce the dental dam to the child as part of the treatment plan.

Index

Quintessentials for General Dental Practitioners Series
in 36 volumes

Editor-in-Chief: Professor Nairn H F Wilson

The Quintessentials for General Dental Practitioners Series covers basic principles and key issues in all aspects of modern dental medicine. Each book can be read as a stand-alone volume or in conjunction with other books in the series.

Publication date, approximately

Oral Surgery and Oral Medicine, Editor: John G Meechan

Practical Dental Local Anaesthesia	available
Practical Oral Medicine	available
Practical Conscious Sedation	available
Practical Surgical Dentistry	Autumn 2005

Imaging, Editor: Keith Horner

Interpreting Dental Radiographs	available
Panoramic Radiology	Autumn 2005
Twenty-first Century Dental Imaging	Spring 2006

Periodontology, Editor: Iain L C Chapple

Understanding Periodontal Diseases: Assessment and Diagnostic Procedures in Practice	available
Decision-Making for the Periodontal Team	available
Successful Periodontal Therapy – A Non-Surgical Approach	available
Periodontal Management of Children, Adolescents and Young Adults	available
Periodontal Medicine: A Window on the Body	Autumn 2005

Implantology, Editor: Lloyd J Searson

Implantology in General Dental Practice	available
Managing Orofacial Pain in Practice	Spring 2006

Endodontics, Editor: John M Whitworth

Rational Root Canal Treatment in Practice	available
Managing Endodontic Failure in Practice	available
Managing Dental Trauma in Practice	Autumn 2005
Preventing Pulpal Injury in Practice	Autumn 2005

Prosthodontics, Editor: P Finbarr Allen

Teeth for Life for Older Adults	available
Complete Dentures – from Planning to Problem Solving	available
Removable Partial Dentures	available
Fixed Prosthodontics in Dental Practice	available
Occlusion: A Theoretical and Team Approach	Spring 2006

Operative Dentistry, Editor: Paul A Brunton

Decision-Making in Operative Dentistry	available
Aesthetic Dentistry	available
Indirect Restorations	Spring 2006
Communicating in Dental Practice: Stress Free Dentistry and Improved Patient Care	Spring 2006
Applied Dental Materials in Operative Dentistry	Spring 2006

Paediatric Dentistry/Orthodontics, Editor: Marie Therese Hosey

Child Taming: How to Cope with Children in Dental Practice	available
Paediatric Cariology	available
Treatment Planning for the Developing Dentition	Autumn 2005

General Dentistry and Practice Management, Editor: Raj Rattan

The Business of Dentistry	available
Risk Management	available
Practice Management for the Dental Team	Autumn 2005
Quality Matters: From Clinical Care to Customer Service	Autumn 2005
Dental Practice Design	Spring 2006
IT in Dentistry: A Working Manual	Spring 2006

Quintessence Publishing Co. Ltd., London